EVERYTHING

YOU NEED TO KNOW ABOUT...

Pilates

EVERYTHING

YOU NEED TO KNOW ABOUT...

Pilates

FOUNDERS OF THE PILATES CENTRE
**AMY TAYLOR ALPERS AND
RACHEL TAYLOR SEGEL**
WITH LORNA GENTRY

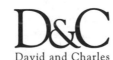

David and Charles

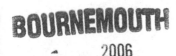
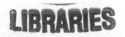

A DAVID & CHARLES BOOK

David & Charles is a subsidiary of F+W (UK) Ltd.,
an F+W Publications Inc. company

First published in the UK in 2005
First published in the USA as The Everything® Pilates Book,
by Adams Media in 2002

A catalogue record for this book is available from the British Library.

ISBN 0 7153 2320 2

Printed in Great Britain by CPI Bath
for David & Charles
Brunel House   Newton Abbot   Devon

Visit our website at www.davidandcharles.co.uk

David & Charles books are available from all good bookshops;
alternatively you can contact our Orderline on (0)1626 334555 or
write to us at FREEPOST EX2110, David & Charles Direct,
Newton Abbot, TQ12 4ZZ (no stamp required UK only).

Contents

Dedication

We dedicate this book to all students and teachers of the Pilates method – past, present and future.

Acknowledgments

We would never have been able to write this book without the help of many important people. We want to thank the following:

Our 'super' models: Debora Kolwey, Lisa Csillan McAleavy, Bryan Meeks and Jonathan Oldham, as well as Jennifer Czech Bergen, Mary Bischof, Frederica Robin Kolwey and Kim Haroche.

Our photographers, Steve Collector and Kate Black; our artist, Len Segel; and our equipment supplier, Peak Body Systems.

Thanks also to the following people: Amy Lange, a gifted Pilates teacher, who read our drafts and gave us invaluable advice; our agent, Kathy Welton; Kevin Bowen and The Pilates Method Alliance; Tom Gordon, Mark Spenard and David Schwartz; and all the patient and supportive staff, clients and trainees of The Pilates Centre, Boulder, Colorado, USA.

Thanks to Daniela Coles, who was consultant for the British edition of this book.

We also want to thank Joe and Clara Pilates and the students they inspired – who in turn inspired us – especially Romana Kryzanowska, who first instilled the love for Pilates in us, and Kathy Grant, who offered her time and memories.

And most of all, we want to thank our wonderful families, whose patience, generosity, constant support and love were essential: Len, Olivia and Eleanor Segel; and Richard, Nathanael and Lily Alpers!

Foreword

As president of the Pilates Method Alliance, I was asked to recommend an author for this project. I did not take this task lightly. Immediately, two people came to my mind. Amy Taylor Alpers and Rachel Taylor Segel are sisters, partners, friends and, above all, Pilates professionals with the highest integrity. They are the owners of the internationally renowned studio and teacher-training facility, The Pilates Centre in Boulder, Colorado, USA.

Amy and Rachel have been quietly and diligently carrying on the Pilates work with the highest integrity for well over ten years. I knew that their enthusiasm, knowledge and attention to detail would help to create a remarkable, high-quality Pilates book that our entire community would be proud to see in print.

Everything You Need to Know about Pilates was created with love by these two remarkable individuals. Enjoy their insights, knowledge and expertise – and may Joe and Clara Pilates be with you as you explore this remarkable system of movement.

In health,

Kevin A. Bowen
President, Pilates Method Alliance

Introduction

Joseph Hubertus Pilates was an extraordinary, outspoken, vibrant person – arguably a genius – who was a man truly driven to help people be healthy. During his 60 or so years of pioneering work in the fitness industry, Joseph Pilates helped thousands of people be healthy, 'be alive', and his exceptional and powerful fitness technique is more popular today than ever.

'Never in history', Joseph Pilates wrote in his book, *Your Health*, 'have more time and money been expended to attain normal physical perfection than in the present era!' He was writing in 1934. Although times have changed dramatically since then, the fitness problems he saw around him haven't changed much at all. People still suffer from too much stress, tend to lead sedentary lives, and all too often try to 'buy' a fast fitness fix or cram their entire fitness programme into a few muscle-wrenching workouts a week.

These are all problems Joseph Pilates wrote about in his 1945 book *Return to Life Through Contrology*, seeking to tell the world about 'Contrology', as Pilates had termed his method. Though this term may have faded from popularity, the fitness programme certainly didn't; today, Contrology is known as the Pilates method – or simply Pilates.

The purpose of this book is to inspire people to be in control of their own health and well-being through the Pilates method. Whether you know nothing about Pilates or are already teaching it professionally, this book has something to offer you. It includes in-depth explanations of eleven quintessential powerful Pilates mat exercises, with detailed step-by-step directions that give you a great workout at home. More important is the book's detailed examination of the Pilates philosophy, fundamental principles and goals sought by all those who want to achieve peak mental and physical health.

The benefits you achieve through this unique and wonderful system of exercise are numerous: a strong, sleek, supple body that breathes deeply and fully, a healthy heart that promotes oxygen-rich blood to flow 'with renewed vigour', and body/mind coordination that uplifts the spirit. In other words, a body 'fully capable of naturally, easily and satisfactorily performing our many and varied daily tasks with spontaneous zest and pleasure', as Pilates himself described it in *Return to Life Through Contrology*, for 'physical fitness is the first prerequisite of happiness'.

This book also includes other important Pilates information: a history of Joseph and Clara Pilates and their primary protégés; a look at all the main pieces of Pilates equipment; a discussion on how to choose a teacher or facility at which to study; advice for setting up a home studio; and even some information on what to wear during your Pilates workout. For those of you who love Pilates already and are thinking of making a career change, we've included a section on becoming an instructor.

Today, Pilates is heavily infused with the personality and strength of the man who created it, and his enthusiasm, delight and commitment speak loudly from these pages. More than 75 years after Joseph Pilates first introduced his amazing system, the Pilates method of fitness conditioning is more popular than ever before, with students from all walks of life and with a wide range of fitness needs and capabilities.

CHAPTER 1

The Powerful Benefits of Pilates

You're interested in Pilates, but you may not understand how powerful a tool this system of movement and exercise can be. Whether you're young or old, an experienced athlete or a novice, this book will help you understand how the Pilates system can make it possible for you to attain your fitness goals.

Understanding the Benefits

Everyone benefits from Pilates in their own unique ways, but Pilates offers a myriad of unchanging, invaluable benefits for everyone, including the following improvements in your physical and mental condition: good circulation; deep, healthy breathing and increased lung capacity; strength and flexibility; healthy bones and joints; improved posture, balance and coordination; a strong abdomen and a powerful 'core'; energy, stamina and stress relief; reduction of body 'aches and pains'; and prevention of reinjury of damaged muscles and joints – the list can go on and on.

Although this may sound too good to be true, Pilates gives you control of your own body and, therefore, your life! And, most important, the benefits of Pilates aren't exclusively for a few die-hard fanatics. With regular practice of this time-proven system at home and in the studio, anyone can experience these and other Pilates benefits.

Energy and Endurance

Regular Pilates practice energizes your body and increases its endurance by improving your strength and flexibility, as well as your breathing, circulation and posture. Proper breathing is central to every Pilates exercise. Joseph Pilates believed that you had to clean your lungs with every breath, completely emptying them of 'stale' air before refilling them. Deep breathing 'oxygenates' your system, sending oxygen coursing through your arteries and throughout all your body tissues.

Joe Pilates referred to vibrant, nourishing blood flow as being the 'equivalent of an internal shower'. He went on to say that his exercises 'purify the blood... with the result that the organs of the body... receive the benefit of clean, fresh blood carried to them by the rejuvenated bloodstream.'

Your ability to feel energized and refreshed, however, requires more than a good set of lungs and a strong heart. If you drag those healthy organs and systems around in a slumped, misaligned body, you won't keep them healthy for long. When you stand erect and strong, you elongate and align your body's framework, and that helps to pull your internal organs in line and give them plenty of room to function as they should. A properly erect stance and seated posture allow your lungs to expand fully. Your abdominal muscles naturally pull in, giving better support to your lower back. Your spine is strong and evenly balances the weight of your body. By directly contributing to your breathing, circulation, carriage, stance and grace of movement, Pilates builds endurance and helps you feel more energetic, relaxed and ready to take on the challenges of the day.

Exceptional Resistance Training

FIGURE 1-1

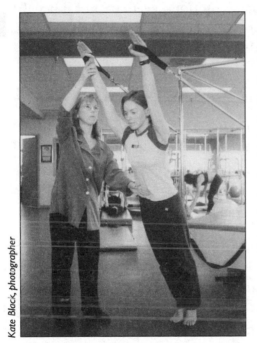

Kate Black, photographer

Nearly all Pilates equipment comes equipped with straps and springs that offer resistance training of a type that is unique to the Pilates method. Resistance training is an important part of many fitness programmes, including Nautilus, weightlifting, rowing, stair-climbing workouts and so on. In those workout techniques, weights and machine pulleys are used to resist the energy of your muscles to increase the workout benefit that those muscles receive.

In Pilates, however, the equipment increases the workout benefit by teaching your muscles to become springs themselves. Pilates designed his equipment to facilitate people in doing movements they can't achieve without assistance.

For instance, the exercise presented in FIGURE 1-1 uses the resistance of the springs to strengthen and 'centre' the body, integrating it into one powerful whole. As strength and control build over time, the Pilates student becomes capable of performing the movements without the aid of the machines.

To understand this effect, imagine you're on roller skates and your legs begin to slide apart. If you had a spring connecting your skates, this would help you draw your legs together. The more often you drew your legs together, the stronger you would become and the less you'd need to rely on the spring. And, if you were conditioned in the Pilates method, not only would you be able to bring your legs back together, but you would have the flexibility, suppleness and control to perform full leg-splits without risking injury.

With or without the equipment, Pilates exercises are designed to utilize your own body as part of your resistance-training programme. Your body acts as both the resistance against which you push and pull, as well as the actual weight you lift and move. As you lift, curl and move your body in the controlled Pilates motions, every part of it benefits from the weightlifting work of that movement. This form of resistance training builds supple strength without unnecessary bulk.

Who Benefits from Pilates?

Many exercise programmes just aren't designed for everyone. Some knees can't handle the pounding workout of a five-mile jog, some elderly joints can't hold the pace of a 45-minute session on a stair machine, and joining a step-aerobics class can feel like jumping aboard a moving goods train to just about anyone who's out of shape.

Pilates is for everyone and everyone benefits from doing the Pilates exercises and movements. If you're a typical professional, office worker or student, for example, you spend a good amount of your time in front of a computer. You sit hunched up and cramped; your breathing grows shallow; and your shoulder and hip muscles tighten as your abdominal muscles sag. Pilates training combats these bad habits by teaching your body to naturally assume a well-aligned, strong position. You learn to breathe deeply, and to use every movement as a controlled exercise in strength and grace.

Pilates is a great way to 'shape up', but the benefits of Pilates go well beyond shedding a few pounds. Pilates training benefits beginners, children, older people, athletes, dancers – just about everybody. It has helped people recover from an injury, fight chronic pain, train for athletic competition and – yes – get into shape.

You Don't Have to Be Fit to Get Fit

Here's the best news about Pilates: you can do it. As Joseph Pilates said, 'If you will faithfully perform your Contrology exercises regularly only four times a week for just three months… you will find your body development approaching the ideal, accompanied by renewed mental vigour and spiritual enhancements.' Joe believed that anyone could look forward to those results, no matter what level of fitness he or she might bring to the first Pilates session.

Pilates is a low-impact exercise, designed to help anyone return to the health they enjoyed when young, and learn to move smoothly and confidently, with strong, uniformly developed muscles and calm, focused energy. If you're out of shape, you can modify Pilates exercises to fit your current ability – in fact, you will learn many of those modifications in this book. You don't have to be strong and healthy to start Pilates – doing it will take you there!

As with any fitness programme, you should always check with your doctor before beginning Pilates training; he or she will know if you have any special physical needs, conditions or injuries that might prohibit you from learning and practising the Pilates exercises.

Pilates Is for Kids

You're never too young to start doing Pilates (see FIGURE 1-2 overleaf). In fact, Joseph Pilates based many Pilates exercises on the movements of babies and children. Pilates saw the 'downhill slide' of the human body beginning at a very early age. He bemoaned the fact that we overdress our children, feed them too often, force artificial rest and play schedules on them, and divert them from the natural, healthy development they should enjoy.

Joe saw little benefit in most contemporary physical education programmes, because they didn't really educate people about fitness. In his opinion, most students of fitness programmes 'are drilled to do stunts for which their bodies are unfit. While their bodies are incorrectly developed, their mental control is absolutely neglected.'

FIGURE 1-2

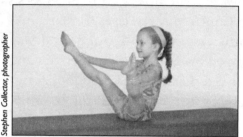

Stephen Collector, photographer

The Pilates method supports natural growth, and the stretching and decompression benefits of Pilates are especially appealing to children: practising Pilates makes them feel tall, strong and self-confident. Because Pilates emphasizes uniform development, children aren't trained to develop one 'pet' muscle group. Instead, all muscles – large and small alike – are developed evenly and concurrently, helping children with overall strength, flexibility and coordination. Because Pilates exercises encourage children to be more aware and in control of their movements, children are better able to develop poise, confidence and balance.

Because Pilates is a disciplined exercise programme, it does pose a special challenge for the young. However, it is a challenge worth tackling: the result of practising Pilates is a good physical and mental foundation for developing skills and interests in sports, dance, gymnastics – and life.

You're Never Too Old

It's wonderful that people are living longer these days, but old age inevitably presents obstacles. Many find that some parts of their bodies tend to outlast the others. Your heart may be strong, but if your joints stop working and become painful and swollen, you may not feel like remaining active, fit and involved with life.

Some people will avoid pain by giving up all of the enjoyable things that used to occupy their lives, but sacrificing enjoyment in the pursuit of a pain-free existence deprives them of much of life's pleasures.

Pilates is one of the greatest tools for keeping ageing bodies . . . well, ageless. It's a method custom-made for slowing the pace at which the body ages, as all the exercises can be readily adapted and modified according to each individual's requirements. Here are just a few of the Pilates benefits that are especially valuable to the middle-aged and older:

· Improvement of your heart, lungs and the rest of the circulatory system.
· Stronger and more resilient bones and joints that 'bounce' instead of breaking.
· Improved balance and coordination, and a newfound sense of confidence in your body.

It's easy to lose your confidence as you age. Suddenly you find you're not very good at doing some of the things you never had to think about before. Regular Pilates practice makes you stronger, more flexible and more confident. You can do more, and you know it.

Many older people fear falling, and with good reason. As you age, your bones become more brittle. At the same time, if your muscles grow weak with age, you become more wobbly, less sure on your feet and more prone to falls. A broken hip, ankle or knee can signal months of painful recovery – and for some, the end of a mobile life. With the right supervision from a qualified instructor, Pilates will help you strengthen your muscles, bones and joints, and will enhance your mind/body connection, all powerful weapons in helping you fight old age.

Pilates Is for Athletes

Pilates is very popular with athletes, and with good reason – it's capable of challenging even professional athletes. A good Pilates instructor teaches Pilates to address the specific needs and capabilities of the individual client, and to challenge and benefit students at any level of fitness. If you're a seasoned trainer or conditioned athlete, the instructor will show you just how much you can gain from regular Pilates practice.

Pilates provides your body with deep overall conditioning, as it elongates, strengthens and aligns your body and balances the inconsistencies resulting from sports-specific training. Many athletes have turned to Pilates as a great cross-training technique to help them improve their bodies. No matter what your sport of choice, Pilates can help you improve in it.

Can I mix Pilates with weight training?
Yes, and weight trainers have particular benefits to draw from Pilates. Many weight-training exercises tend to concentrate on isolated muscle groups, where the muscles 'bulk up' over time. Pilates simultaneously strengthens and lengthens your muscles uniformly, creating supple power.

Remember, Pilates works your entire body uniformly – something that few traditional sports (or exercise programmes) are designed to do. Many sports develop the body asymmetrically, as when tennis players and golfers develop a strong 'forward' arm. Pilates balances the body's development, which is important for a number of reasons, including the following:

· Increased overall body strength, endurance, balance and coordination.
· Uniformly developed muscle groups that promote efficient and productive muscle movement. You get more sustained muscle growth and development from every movement when you develop all muscle groups uniformly.

Pilates corrects muscular imbalances, such as tight hamstrings, overloaded quads or overstretched lower backs, caused by running, skiing, cycling and other sports. In addition to improving coordination, control, balance, precision, endurance, breathing capacity and efficient movement patterns, Pilates also prevents and helps rehabilitate sports injuries.

Walkers, runners, skiers, scuba divers, golfers, cricket players, gymnasts, boxers – you'll find people who have benefited from Pilates in the ranks of nearly every organized athletic group. Tennis champion Pat Cash, Olympic rowing Gold medallist Matthew Pinsent and former

England cricket captain Mike Atherton – not to mention the English National Ballet – have all turned to Pilates to stretch and strengthen muscles, build endurance and develop balanced, uniform bodies. The Pilates method also teaches the technique of visualization, which nearly all athletes use to achieve peak athletic performance.

The Pilates/Dance Connection

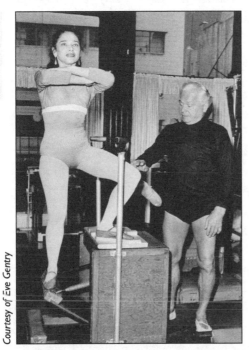

FIGURE 1-3:
Joseph Pilates with Eve Gentry

Courtesy of Eve Gentry

Pilates himself was not a dancer, nor did he develop his method specifically with dancers in mind. However, dancers were among the first professional 'athletes' to turn to Pilates for fitness and injury rehabilitation. Early dance pioneers such as Martha Graham and George Balanchine appreciated the strengthening and lengthening benefits of Pilates training, and many of their students trained with Joe and his wife, Clara. All five of the first-generation Pilates master teachers – Romana Kryzanowska, Eve Gentry, Kathy Grant, Ron Fletcher and Carola Trier – were dancers who came to Joe for help with injury rehabilitation.

In New York City, thousands of dancers passed through the Pilates studio, and Pilates remains a favourite physical training and rehabilitation technique for dancers around the world. In the UK, Pilates exercises are taught at dance conservatories and in Higher Education dance programmes up and down the country, including the Laban Centre, London, University College, Chichester, Middlesex University, The Place, London, and the University of Surrey, Roehampton.

The benefits of Pilates aren't limited to ballet. Flamenco, jazz, chorus-line and tap dancers, as well as ballroom dancers, have benefited from the flexibility, strength, alignment, balance, strong posture and graceful, flowing movement that they gain through regular Pilates practice.

Pilates helps dancers improve their concentration, their dance technique and form, and their muscular control, strength, balance and coordination. In February 1956, an article in *Dance* magazine reported, 'At some time or other, virtually every dancer in New York... has meekly submitted to the spirited instruction of Joe Pilates.'

Reaping the Mind/Body Benefits of Pilates

When Joseph Pilates wrote *Your Health* (1934), he offered the Western world some rather surprising opinions on fitness. Pilates believed that good health requires balanced fitness of body and mind, and that you can't develop your body without developing your mind as well – an approach similar to those found in Eastern fitness traditions. To that end, Pilates encouraged his students to actively engage their minds in every movement and exercise they performed.

For example, because the Pilates method emphasizes controlled breathing, you have to focus your concentration on each breath, paying close attention to the expansion and contraction of your lungs, and the way your chest, diaphragm and abdomen move during breathing. As you learn correct breathing techniques, your body adopts better breathing as its natural method, and you no longer have to 'tell' your lungs how to do their job.

Visualization and Imagination

Visualization and imagination are important tools in following the Pilates method. In fact, many consider visualization to be as essential to a good Pilates workout as the Pilates exercises and equipment. Many instructors use visualization to help students 'feel' their way into new movements and exercises, and to override deeply ingrained patterns and habits. Regular Pilates practice gives you a new awareness of your body and its capabilities. You learn to stand, sit and move with purpose and grace. Your balance and coordination improve as your mind and body work together to give you a firm, sure step and a strong, upright body. Your mind is your body's best partner, and Pilates helps you build a truly successful mind/body partnership.

To experience visualization at work, try the following exercise: pull your stomach in, notice how that feels, then release your stomach muscles. Now imagine that your stomach is sliding in and up, massaging the front of your spine. Note the difference in the quality of sensation. This visualization of your stomach's movement gives the experience a lifting, lengthening quality.

Using Pilates to Relieve Stress

As Joe Pilates stated in *Return to Life Through Contrology* (1945), his fitness 'develops the body uniformly, corrects wrong postures, restores physical vitality, invigorates the mind and elevates the spirit'. Stress relief is a major result of achieving all of those goals.

Stress frequently 'collects' in the neck and shoulders, tightening muscles and pulling shoulders in and up. Pilates lengthens your neck and spine, and this open, erect posture helps release tension in your head, neck and shoulders, enabling you to breathe more deeply and fully.

Many people begin Pilates practice strictly for stress reduction. Those suffering from hypertension and chronic fatigue often find that the Pilates approach to controlled breath and deep, lengthening movement relaxes and refreshes their bodies.

Pilates Is an Overall Fitness Programme

Regular Pilates practice is one of the best overall fitness tools you can use. Elizabeth Hurley, Glenn Close, Madonna, Sarah Ferguson and Vidal

Sassoon, along with an uncounted number of supermodels, actors and entertainers, have turned to Pilates to firm themselves up, get fit and get in shape. Pilates builds a sleek, slim body, and it's especially noted for developing a strong, flat abdomen.

But Pilates fitness goes beyond the fitting room. By retraining your body to walk, sit, stand and move correctly, Pilates turns every movement into a mini-fitness session. Pilates makes you feel better in everything you do and makes you taller, too.

A Programme for a Lifetime

One of the most important aspects of any general fitness programme is its ability to meet your needs over a period of time. It's easy to lose interest in many fitness programmes, to become bored with their repetitive and unchanging rituals – to 'fall out of love' with a particular sport and stop practising it.

Whether jogging or working out at the gym, your biggest goal in any fitness programme is to make it into a habit, and Pilates is an easy habit to fall into. It's a non-competitive practice based on natural movements, so it offers a refreshing change from the typical 'no-pain-no-gain-feel-the-burn' workout mentality. Moreover, Pilates requires mental focus that keeps you intrigued and personally involved in your activity; it offers a wide variety of movements, exercises and routines that keep sessions fresh, challenging and fun, so it's anything but mindless or boring. Pilates practice will leave you feeling energized, refreshed and relaxed – not drained and exhausted.

A good Pilates instructor is an invaluable aid in learning and mastering the full range of Pilates exercises. However, you're the one in charge of your Pilates fitness programme. True to its original name, Contrology, Pilates teaches and demands 'control'; you control your fitness programme, progress and ultimate success.

Because Pilates is adaptable to any fitness level, it will allow you to gradually build your body's strength, flexibility and endurance, proceeding at your own pace. As your body changes and its fitness needs evolve, your Pilates programme can be adapted to these changes. Pilates puts you so closely in contact with your body and its condition that you will know what your body needs to do, what it's capable of doing, and what you should avoid.

Because Pilates movements and exercises create uniform development – balancing, strengthening and lengthening all the muscles with each exercise – Pilates is actually a more efficient way to work out. No need to spend an hour warming up, stretching and getting your heart pumping, then another hour lifting weights. Pilates works all the muscles all the time. If overall fitness is your goal, Pilates is your ticket for getting there.

Pilates helps your body stay young, fit and full of vitality. As Joe himself once said, in *Return to Life Through Contrology*, 'With body, mind and spirit functioning perfectly as a coordinated whole, what else could reasonably be expected, other than an active, alert, disciplined person?'

CHAPTER 2

Joseph Pilates and His Protégés: A Short History

Joseph Pilates was a pioneer in the Western world's fitness movement and the creator of the Pilates method, which he originally called 'Contrology'. This chapter examines the history of the Pilates movement, to give you a clear picture of how Pilates became the popular fitness programme of today.

The Story of Joseph Pilates

FIGURE 2-1:
Joseph Pilates

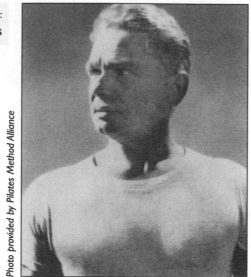

Photo provided by Pilates Method Alliance

Even as a child, Joseph Pilates was captivated by the human body's potential for natural, healthy movement. According to an article by Evelyn Ringold in the *New York Herald Tribune*, he would spend hours studying anatomy books, 'learning every page, every part of the body; I would move each part as I memorized it. As a child, I would lie in the woods for hours, hiding and watching the animals move.' As he said at the age of 86, 'I must be right. Never an aspirin. Never sick a day in my life. The whole country, the whole world should do my exercises. They'd be happier.' Here is the story of how Joseph Pilates developed his popular fitness programme.

Joe's Early Years

Joseph Pilates was born in München-Glebach, a small village near Düsseldorf, Germany, in 1880. His father was a prize-winning gymnast and his mother was a naturopath. In his early childhood, Joseph was plagued with illnesses such as asthma, rickets and rheumatic fever, and was often teased because he was so frail. These factors helped develop his commitment to improving his fitness and health.

At a very young age, Joseph began working to build his physical strength and stamina; by the age of 14, he was in such prime physical condition that he was used as a model for a series of illustrated anatomical charts (these charts would hang in his New York studio decades later). Joe was a self-taught athlete who eventually excelled at skiing, diving, gymnastics and boxing.

Pilates Begins His Work
in Fitness and Rehabilitation

In 1912, Joe came to England. Reports vary on why he came here or what he did; some say he went to train as a boxer, while others claim that he and his brother toured England with a German circus troupe, doing a Greek statue act. In any event, when World War I erupted in 1914, Joseph's German heritage made him an enemy alien in England and he was placed in an internment camp, first in Lancaster and later on the Isle of Man. Joe's confinement evidently didn't dampen his spirits; before long, he was teaching his fellow internees wrestling and self-defence, and his skills in fitness training soon led to work with the camp's disabled.

Joe began assisting the camp's hospital in helping bedridden patients regain strength and muscle control. To assist these people in their exercises, Joe adapted hospital beds with pulleys, straps and springs. As he later said, 'I thought, why use my strength? So I made a machine to do it for me.' These adapted beds were the forerunners of the Pilates exercise equipment used today.

Joe often proudly stated that during the raging influenza pandemic that swept the world in 1918, none of the people he worked with at the Isle of Man camp contracted the flu. Tens of millions of healthy young people died from this virulent strain of flu, particularly the incarcerated populations, so Joe had good reason to be proud of this success.

After the war, he returned to Germany, eventually settling in Hamburg, where he continued developing his fitness theories and exercises, and spreading the word about his techniques. The Hamburg Military Police became aware of Joe's work, and hired him as the department's self-defence and physical fitness trainer.

During this time, several important movement innovators worked with Joe Pilates. Rudolph von Laban, a noted dance choreographer and movement analyst, observed Pilates' body conditioning methods and movements and incorporated some of Joe's theories and exercises into his own work, as did the German dancer/choreographers Mary Wigman and Hanya Holm.

By 1925, Joseph Pilates had achieved a certain fame, which brought him to the attention of the German government. When the German government asked him to train the new German army, Pilates realized that the changing political climate might compromise his ability to pursue his own path with his work. Joseph Pilates decided to take his dream – and his skills – to a new homeland, and he set sail for America.

The First Pilates Studio

On the ship that took Joseph Pilates to the United States, he encountered a quiet kindergarten teacher and nurse named Clara. By all accounts, Clara was smitten with Joe's warm personality and enthusiasm for life, and they eventually married. Reports say that Pilates devised a series of rehabilitative exercises that relieved her arthritis pain. They opened their first studio at 939 Eighth Avenue shortly after they arrived in New York City in 1926.

The Pilates's studio shared a building with several New York dance organizations, and it didn't take long for the dancers to discover Joe. Pilates's fame spread throughout the dance community; George Balanchine encouraged his dancers to follow the Pilates exercise programme, as did Martha Graham, Jerome Robbins and Ted Shawn. In addition, in the summers from 1939 to 1951 Joe and Clara went to teach at Jacobs Pillow, a well-known dance camp in the Berkshire Mountains. Over the years, dancers came to rely on Pilates training techniques for both fitness and rehabilitation.

Pilates didn't train just dancers. His studio soon became *the* fitness centre of New York City, drawing a number of the city's richest and most influential citizens, including Columbia University president Chester Bowles, Katharine Hepburn, Sir Laurence Olivier, Yehudi Menuhin, Mrs Jean Vanderbilt and – to quote a newspaper article from 1964 – 'prominent New Yorkers named Guggenheim and Gimbel'. All these people trekked to Pilates' studio, to be led through mat work and equipment exercises by Joe and Clara.

FIGURE 2-2:
Joseph
Pilates at 57

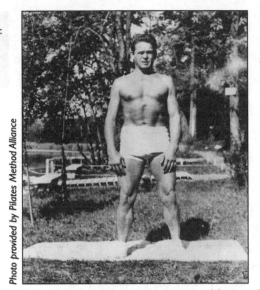

Photo provided by Pilates Method Alliance

Pilates taught in his studio through the late 1960s. During these years, Joe continued to be healthy and vibrant, teaching students, talking with reporters and jogging through Manhattan in his bathing suit. In 1956, a *Dance* magazine writer described the 76-year-old Pilates as follows: 'A stocky 175 pounds, with bristling gray hair and pale, child-like blue eyes, he bounces about, pushing here, punching there, like a middleweight fighter skirmishing in the ring.'

Joseph Pilates maintained his unbelievably robust health until the end of his life. In 1966, a fire hit the Eighth Avenue building, damaging the back rooms of the facility, where Joe rented some storage space. According to Bruce King, a longtime Pilates student and teacher who lived in the back of the building, when Joe went back to inspect the damage to his storage room, the burnt floorboards gave out from beneath him. Joe fell through the floor, but was able to catch hold of one of the floor beams and pull himself out of danger – no small feat, when you consider that Pilates was nearly 86 years old at the time.

Joe didn't lead a monk's life, either. Over beer, steak and a cigar, he exclaimed to one reporter, 'I eat what I feel like eating. If people could see the way I live – smoking, drinking and loving – they wouldn't believe it. Loving! Without it you are dead!'

But Pilates was not immortal; he died the next year, at the age of 87. According to some sources, the cause of death might have been complications due to smoke inhalation suffered during the fire. Clara continued her work at the studio, teaching the Pilates method of fitness after Joe's death. In 1971, when she was ready for retirement, Clara turned over the Pilates studio to a trusted and experienced Pilates student and instructor, Romana Kryzanowska. Although Clara's teaching days were over, she continued visiting the studio in its new location at 29 West 56th Street, until her death in 1977.

The Pilates Name Goes to Court

When Joseph Pilates died, he left no legally designated heir to the Pilates name and studio practice. When Clara turned the studio over to Romana Kryzanowska in 1971, the business was incorporated and moved to a new location. Over the years, the Pilates studio went through a series of owners, but Ms Kryzanowska remained its director.

Pilates was introduced into the UK by Alan Herdman, who established a successful studio in London in the early 1970s.

In the 1980s, attempts were made to trademark the Pilates name; in 1996, these attempts resulted in a class-action lawsuit that challenged the right of any individual to claim ownership to the use of the Pilates name in connection with the teaching of a method of fitness and body conditioning. In October 2000, a Manhattan federal district court ruled that Pilates is an exercise technique (such as yoga or karate), and therefore the name Pilates cannot be trademarked or restricted by any single entity.

What Does This Mean to You?

Of late you may have read a lot about Pilates, and perhaps you've seen many new Pilates facilities listed in your local Yellow Pages. The overturning of the trademark attempt has been responsible for the plethora of Pilates information and options you see today – videos, articles, books, equipment and studios. Now, instructors are free to say that they are teaching Pilates, and books can freely proclaim that they hold information about the Pilates method of fitness. This is definitely a good thing – but with a few potentially negative consequences.

Because the name Pilates is in the public domain, anyone – and that means anyone – can claim to be teaching the Pilates techniques. With its ever-growing popularity and no overseeing organization to control its name, Pilates is a prime candidate for pirating. That means you have to be a smart Pilates consumer.

In the UK, Skills Active is the Sector Skills Council for Active Leisure and Learning, with the responsibility of raising the skills and qualification levels in the sport, recreation and fitness industries. The recently implemented Register of Exercise Professionals (REPS) is enhancing the confidence of the medical profession and members of the public in the teaching abilities of those working in the industry.

Currently, the major Pilates organizations and training providers are involved in a process with Skills Active to create a National Occupational Standard for Pilates; at time of writing, it is proposed that Pilates will be a category of registration of Level 3 on REPS. Once the National Standard for Pilates has been finalized, a system will be implemented where training organizations can achieve recognition to give entry to REPS. For further information, contact www.skillsactive.com, www.exerciseregister. org, or phone the Development Officer at Skills Active on 0207 632 2000.

Joe's Legacy Lives On

Thanks to some of Joe and Clara's dedicated students, such as Romana Kryzanowska, Carola Trier, Eve Gentry, Kathy Grant and Ron Fletcher, Joe Pilates's methods have survived the decades. Only three first-generation teachers are alive today – Kryzanowska, Fletcher and Grant. Ms Kryzanowska continues to teach Pilates in the New York studio and in seminars around the world. The other teachers established their own studios and continued to develop individual interpretations of the original methods and techniques.

Joe continually developed his movements, exercises and equipment over the course of his lifetime and, consequently, he taught many different variations to different students at different times. This evolutionary process helped to contribute to the many 'schools' of Pilates that exist worldwide today.

When you choose a Pilates instructor or facility, you'll find it helpful to understand which 'school' of instruction your trainer is associated with. This section discusses the primary first-generation instructors – often referred to as the 'Pilates Elders'.

Romana Kryzanowska

Romana Kryzanowska grew up in the Florida Everglades and moved to New York City at an early age to study dance. She became a student at the School of American Ballet, and was introduced to Joseph Pilates in the early 1940s by the school's director, George Balanchine. Kryzanowska had suffered an ankle injury, and Balanchine was hoping that Pilates's fitness conditioning therapy could help her return to dancing.

Sports medicine was unheard of at that time, and Pilates's therapy was one of the few non-surgical treatments available. Joe told Romana, 'If I haven't cured your ankle in five sessions, I'll give you your money back.' Kryzanowska felt improvement in her ankle in just three sessions, and she became a convert to the Pilates philosophy, which became her lifelong practice.

Ms Kryzanowska eventually left New York and moved to Peru, where she lived for over 14 years with her husband and two children. Romana later returned to New York and to Joe's, where he again helped her rehabilitate a knee injury she suffered when she fell into an open manhole while carrying her baby. Romana began teaching Pilates, and – as mentioned earlier in this chapter – eventually was chosen by Clara to take over the operation of the Pilates studio in 1971. The New York studio moved locations twice, and Kryzanowska continued to run it until it closed in 1989, at which point she went on to open her own studio space within Drago's Gym in New York City, where she still teaches today.

Ms Kryzanowska's commitment has always been to maintain the integrity of the original work as it was created and developed by Joseph Pilates. She believes that if you change Pilates's work, you should rename it after yourself instead of continuing to call it Pilates. For years, she has been instructing and certifying others in what many refer to as the 'true' classical Pilates method, and many of her students (including the co-authors of this book) have gone on to open studios of their own.

Kryzanowska is credited with keeping alive Joseph Pilates's original techniques and philosophy.

Ron Fletcher

Ron Fletcher grew up in Missouri, and moved to New York City in 1944. According to his biography, Ron was drawn to dance soon after moving to the city, and in a relatively short time, he became a member of the Martha Graham Dance Company.

> Ron's work today, is – in his words – 'a marvellous organic recipe', flavoured with the teachings of dance masters Martha Graham, Gertrude Shurr and Yeichi Nimura, as well as the techniques of Joseph Pilates. Today, Ron continues to present his workshops, and many instructors who are certified in his technique teach in courses and Pilates facilities around the world.

Fletcher began working with Joe and Clara Pilates after a knee injury sidelined him early in his career. As Ron describes it, Pilates put him to work on the Universal Reformer – an evolutionary heir to those early bedspring-and-frame adaptations Joe designed in the prison-camp hospital during World War I. The Reformer allowed Fletcher to avoid undue pressure on his knee while focusing therapeutic strengthening and lengthening exercises on the surrounding muscles.

Fletcher was able to return to dance and continued his work with the Graham Company. By the 1960s, however, alcohol began to take a toll on his health and career. Fletcher began attending Alcoholics Anonymous, and returned to work with Joe and Clara Pilates in 1967. Joe died later that year, but Fletcher's work with Clara continued.

In 1971, with Clara's blessing, Fletcher opened the Ron Fletcher Studio for Body Contrology on the corner of Wilshire Boulevard and Rodeo Drive in Beverly Hills. At that time, the fitness studio movement was in its infancy. Fletcher's studio offered individual training and personal attention. His approach and the studio's location drew many of

Hollywood's elite, and soon he counted Judith Krantz, Candice Bergen, Ali MacGraw, Dyan Cannon and Barbara Streisand among his clientele.

By the early 1980s, Fletcher began training instructors and certifying individuals in the Ron Fletcher Work and Body Contrology. In addition to teaching Pilates's mat work and equipment exercises, Ron developed a number of new floor-based adaptations of Pilates's equipment exercises, and other techniques he calls 'Towel Work' and 'Percussive Breathing'.

Eve Gentry

Eve Gentry was a master of modern dance and movement who worked with Joseph Pilates for over 20 years. She was also a student of dance master Hanya Holm and motion study expert Rudolph von Laban (who had observed Pilates at work back in Germany prior to World War II).

As a lead dancer with Holm's company, Eve danced up to ten hours a day. Inevitably, the work took its toll, and Eve developed knee and back pain. Hanya Holm then introduced Eve to Joseph Pilates, who began working with her. In a 1994 *Pilates Forum* article, Eve was quoted as saying, 'I'll never forget this sensation – after Joe had worked with me, all of my pains were gone, back pains and knees – everything. It was the first time in three years that I had not had pain, and I felt wonderful.' By 1945, Eve had formed the Eve Gentry Dancers, and she was also teaching at the Pilates's studio.

Based on her work with these masters, Eve developed her own body conditioning technique. In 1968, Eve and her husband, Bruce, opened the Pilates Method Studio in Santa Fe, New Mexico. There she developed a strong rehabilitation practice in addition to training a number of today's top Pilates instructors, including Michelle Larsson and Debora Robinson Kolwey. In 1991, Eve helped found the Institute for the Pilates Method, to carry on the teachings of Joseph Pilates. She continued teaching workshops and teacher training seminars in the Pilates method until shortly before her death in 1994 at the age of 84.

Carola Trier

Joseph Pilates actually helped Carola Trier open her own New York studio in the late 1950s. Carola, a professional dancer and acrobatic contortionist (who performed on roller skates, no less), began studying with Joe in the early 1940s after injuring her back. Her injury was so severe that she thought she'd be using an orthopaedic support for the rest of her life, but after she began working with Pilates, she regained her strength and stability – and found a new mission in life.

Like Joseph Pilates, Carola Trier was born in Germany. She began studying dance and movement as a child, eventually working with Rudolph von Laban at the Folkwang School in Essen. And again like Joe, Carola found Germany an uninviting home for her work in the years preceding World War II. After living in France, she sailed for the USA in 1942. She continued her acrobatic performances in the States until her back injury took her to the studio of Joe and Clara Pilates.

After her own rehabilitation, Carola went on to teach the Pilates method in dance and movement classes around New York City, before opening her own studio on West 58th Street. (A number of the other first-generation teachers taught at Carola's studio early in their teaching careers.)

Carola stressed Pilates's philosophy that uniform development was a key to fitness. She identified common problems in dancers, such as a swaybacked stance, rolled-in feet and hyperextended knees, and developed many Pilates-based exercises to correct these problems. She studied anatomy at Lennox Hill Hospital; Dr Jordan, who worked at Lennox Hill, began to send his patients to her for rehabilitation. Carola continued teaching Pilates until the mid-1980s; she died in 2000, at the age of 87.

Some of Carola's best-known students are the dancers Brenda Anderson and Mary Kasakove (who taught for Carola for 18 years), Fran Lehen (author of *How to Improve Your Posture*) and Jillian Hessel, who operates her own Pilates studio in California. Another of Carola's successful students, Deborah Lessen, owns the Green Street Studio in New York City and is a founding board member of the Pilates Method Alliance.

Kathy Grant

Kathleen Stanford Grant is another important keeper of the Pilates flame. Like many of Joe's students, Kathy Grant was a dancer before she began her training in Pilates. As a child in the late 1920s, she studied at the Boston Conservatory of Music. She was a chorus girl at New York's famous Zanzibar Club, and worked in a number of Broadway and off-Broadway productions and television programmes, and toured in the United States, Europe, Africa and the Middle East. Kathy also worked as a choreographer and co-director for a number of dance companies, and helped choreograph the 1984 film *Cotton Club*. She also worked closely with Arthur Mitchell, the founder of the Dance Theatre of Harlem.

Kathy Grant was introduced to Joe Pilates by Pearl Lang, a well-known dancer. Kathy had injured her knee in a fall, and was hoping that Pilates could help her rehabilitate her knee so she could return to dancing. Kathy Grant became a longtime student of Joe Pilates, and she was one of only two people to receive official Pilates certification through a federally subsidized programme of instruction approved of and supervised by Joe himself at the New York State Division of Vocational Rehabilitation. (Lolita San Miguel, director of Ballet Concierto de Puerto Rico, was the other.)

Kathy taught at Carola Trier's studio and later managed the Pilates studio in the famous Henri Bendel department store from 1972 until it closed in 1988. Joe had opened that studio in 1965, to offer his training techniques in the store's highly fashionable beauty salon. After the studio closed, Kathy continued teaching Pilates in workshops and seminars around the world. Today, Kathy Grant continues to teach Pilates on the faculty of the Department of Dance at the Tisch School of the Arts, New York University.

Fifty Years Ahead of His Time

During his lifetime, Joseph Pilates did not receive the exposure and recognition he so richly deserved. As the sole creator and source of his life's work, he focused his genius on developing his method, and consequently was able to train only a select handful of students to carry on his teachings. 'What I need is a school where I can turn out other teachers', he stated in 1946. Today, his dream is finally being realized.

'The acquirement and enjoyment of physical well-being, mental calm and spiritual peace are priceless to their possessors... [and] it is only through Contrology that this unique trinity of a balanced body, mind and spirit can ever be attained.'

Joseph Pilates, *Return to Life Through Contrology*

CHAPTER 3

The Fundamentals of Pilates

In describing his method of body conditioning and fitness training, Joseph Pilates covered a wide range of issues, offering his students advice on every aspect of daily life, from proper diet to the correct technique for showering! No matter how broad its range of suggested techniques is, however, the Pilates method is firmly founded on certain principles and goals.

The Guiding Principles of Pilates

Joseph Pilates developed his fitness method with one overriding goal: to give people a way to achieve 'true health'. He defined true health as 'the attainment and maintenance of a uniformly developed body' with a well-balanced 'holy trinity' of body, mind and spirit. The guiding principles described in this chapter are fundamental to learning and practising the Pilates method.

More importantly, you will follow these principles to achieve the fundamental Pilates goals of uniform development, deep healthy breathing, flexible and decompressed spine and joints, robust circulation and the trinity of body/mind/spirit.

Concentration and Awareness

Concentration and awareness are like the macro and micro focus functions of a single lens – you need both to be able to concentrate on the specifics and be aware of the whole. Concentration enables you to make precise controlled movements. To do any Pilates movement or exercise correctly, you must be able to focus your attention and intense concentration on certain body parts or specific skills. Every single movement matters.

Maintaining awareness means paying attention to your entire body – knowing what all the parts of your body are doing at any given moment; it means being aware of your muscles, your body position, your breathing, the way the movement feels, and how your joints and muscles respond to each repetition.

Heightened awareness is one of the skills that helps Pilates clients have more balance and coordination; because they're aware of their bodies in space and their surroundings, they move with confidence and security, without fear of stumbling, running into objects or in other ways injuring themselves. Awareness facilitates your movement with grace, stability and harmony with your surroundings.

As you become adept at doing Pilates with concentration and awareness, your mind tracks each movement. Here is what a typical thought process of somebody doing Pilates might sound like:

> This movement begins here; when I extend my leg, my abdomen draws in, massaging my spine; my ankle is flexed, and now I need to point it; as I lower my leg I really need to rescoop my abdominals to stabilize my spine while I squeeze every atom of air out of my lungs.

Awareness makes you 'present' in every Pilates movement and exercise. In the course of any series of Pilates movements, your body is in a continual state of evolution. With each succeeding repetition, your muscles become more responsive, your joints become more flexible and so on. Being present in your workout enables you to sense the changes and continue to challenge and develop your body in new ways with each movement repetition.

When you repeat a movement, therefore, you are using a new, evolved body. As a result, each repetition is a new experience, rather than a remembered response. As tight places open up, weak places grow strong, breathing capacity expands, your mind awakens, and your body and mind respond with movements subtly adapted to do more and get more from each subsequent repetition. There's no better way to know your body than to really notice everything it does.

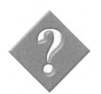

Practising concentration and awareness is difficult – is it necessary?
It is quite difficult to learn, but it's quite simple to do. If you put forth an effort to concentrate your mind on each of your movements, in time you automatically 'read' your entire body and surroundings simultaneously, making you more alert and in control.

In the process of mastering Pilates, you develop your mind to remain constantly aware of and open to your evolving body, mind and spirit, and to the evolving nature, process and results of Pilates movements. The principle of awareness is one of the unique concepts that makes Pilates such a vibrant fitness technique – one that becomes ever more effective over time. The concentration and awareness that guide your Pilates practice eventually become natural and require little effort.

Imagery and Visualization

Concentration and awareness allow you to use your mind creatively through the process of visualization as you do your workout. Visualization is an important part of any Pilates session. Using visualization, you remain aware of and concentrated on your movements and surroundings as you draw upon mental images to help you achieve the exercises' movements and positions. In this way, you are able to experience each repetition anew.

You might imagine, for example, that your spine rolls like a wheel when you do the Roll-Up, or that your spine stretches upwards as though attached to the ceiling by a rubber cord when you do the Spine Stretch. Pilates is a mental and physical workout, and when you do it right, it's engaging, satisfying and never boring.

Using Your Powerhouse

Pilates designated the area of the torso between the lower ribs and hips as the 'Powerhouse' or centre. He believed that correctly developing this area of the body is crucial to mastering his method of body conditioning, and thereby achieving health. A strong Powerhouse forms the foundation for all Pilates movements; energy emanates from the centre and flows out towards your hands and feet. This principle is referred to as 'centring'.

Building and maintaining a strong centre is essential to the Pilates method, and for good health in general, and there are many reasons for this:

- A strong centre supports and decompresses your spine, thereby enabling healthy, graceful movement and providing a natural 'corset' for your vital organs.
- A strong centre promotes proper breathing because it enables you to fully expand and deflate your lungs.
- A strong centre gives you more energy overall, because generating each movement from your centre makes all your movements more efficient.
- A strong centre gives you better control over all of your movements, which in turn improves your posture, poise, grace and balance.

If you've ever practised yoga or other mind/body disciplines, you've used the concept of centring to draw your attention and focus to a single point, to 'stop the internal dialogue' and block out all outside stimuli. For the purposes of this book, the term 'centring' is used to refer to a physical process, although the concept of centring your mind applies to Pilates as well.

Precise Control

Disciplined, precise, controlled movements are hallmarks of the Pilates method. Pilates originally named his method 'Contrology' because he believed that you could become fit and healthy only if you trained your mind to control the actions of your body.

Following your teacher's directions and your own internal motivations is a very important part of the precise control principle. When you study with a Pilates instructor, that person will teach you a very specific set of movements and steps for each Pilates exercise. When you read the exercise instructions in this book, you'll note that each movement is described specifically, carefully and completely. When you perform any Pilates movement, you must exercise precise control to execute the movement exactly as it is meant to be done.

This need for precise control isn't a dogmatic demand for obedience. Every Pilates exercise is designed to provide a very specific benefit. You guide your movements with that benefit in mind – as mentioned earlier, every movement matters. By performing the movement exactly as you're taught to do it, for the specific number of repetitions you're advised to do, you gain the most benefit from the exercise.

To perform a Pilates exercise with precise control, it may be necessary to modify it to your particular capabilities. In Chapters 8–19, you will learn a number of Pilates mat-work exercises, along with modifications to help you perform them with precise control.

There are several important benefits of practising precise control:

· It teaches your muscles to respond precisely to your mind, so that each movement provides the maximum benefit for each muscle group. When you consciously control your muscle movements, you strengthen weak muscles, elongate tight muscles and release tension in overworked muscles, thereby promoting uniform development.
· It works together with the concept of awareness to help you avoid injury. You're more stable and sound on your feet, so you're less likely to trip, move too quickly or bump into things; it will help you avoid injuries that can result from accidentally overextending or overusing joints and muscles.
· It helps discipline your body to the Pilates postures, movements and breathing techniques, giving your body a deeper, more effective workout with every movement you make.

Learning controlled movement gives you much more physical freedom because it enables you to know what your body is (and isn't) capable of doing. Your mind and body will work in such close coordination that you will know when any part of your body has reached its limit.

Flowing Natural Movement

Every Pilates exercise is made up of a series of smooth, fluid movements; you never see a Pilates student strain or jerk to achieve a correct position or movement. The whole-body approach of Pilates fosters connected, graceful, natural movement.

Once you have mastered the basic movements, you don't stop and start and you don't move too quickly or too slowly. You maintain a strong, controlled pace that takes you smoothly through the process of one movement and on to the next. And you carefully coordinate all of your movements with your breathing, to give them even more grace, strength and connected flow.

As you move from exercise to exercise, you make each transition with the same kind of controlled, flowing movement. Because your natural, daily activities involve many transitions, the principle of flowing movement is a valuable one to practise. Remember, Pilates is a re-education of your body and mind.

Flowing, natural movements are safe movements. Any athlete will tell you that controlled, graceful, connected movements are less apt to strain muscles, snap tendons and damage joints.

Classical Advanced Mat Pilates instructors place special emphasis on the connecting transitional movements between exercises. They teach you to move in and out of positions, and to move carefully and thoughtfully whenever you shift your weight or change your posture. This way, your body is prepared to provide the stable support necessary to assume any position. You're more confident, more graceful – and less prone to injury.

Oppositional Energy

Oppositional energy is a principle that combines the skills of concentration and visualization to increase the benefits of movement. Using this principle, you visualize that two opposing points in your body are actually stretching apart as you assume a position or movement, and your muscles react to that visualization by exerting energy in opposing directions. You 'think' the stretch, then your muscles respond to it.

Oppositional energy helps your body refine its physical placement and creates elongation by giving your muscles and joints a mental road map. In Pilates, you use oppositional energy to elongate your spine and decompress all joints – an important goal. Oppositional energy elongates muscles, aligns bones, and balances and stabilizes the muscular forces around each joint. It also gives muscles a deeper workout by adding internal resistance to each muscle group's load.

Oppositional energy helps work all muscle groups simultaneously, by engaging both the muscles used for lengthening and the opposing muscles used to stabilize or resist that pull. For instance, to lengthen and properly position your leg while keeping your pelvis square and stable, you don't want to just push out with your foot. That action might pull your pelvis forward and tilt your body position. Instead, visualize that your hip and heel are actually pulling apart with oppositional energy. This visualization helps you accomplish the stretch without destabilizing the position of your pelvis.

To understand this concept further, sit in a chair and press your sitz bones into the seat as you stretch the top of your head for the ceiling. Notice that every muscle that surrounds your torso – your abdominals and back muscles – automatically responds, balancing, supporting and lifting your upper body. (The use of oppositional energy is also present in the Pilates exercise illustrated in FIGURE 3-1.)

What are sitz bones?
Sitz bones are the part of your pelvis that you sit on; you can find them by sitting on a hard surface and rocking your pelvis back and forth; the bones you feel moving back and forth are your sitz bones.

Oppositional energy automatically engages your centre or Powerhouse, simultaneously and effectively stabilizing, strengthening and decompressing your spinal joints within that suspension force. You feel taller, stronger and more alive. Doesn't that feel great?

FIGURE 3-1

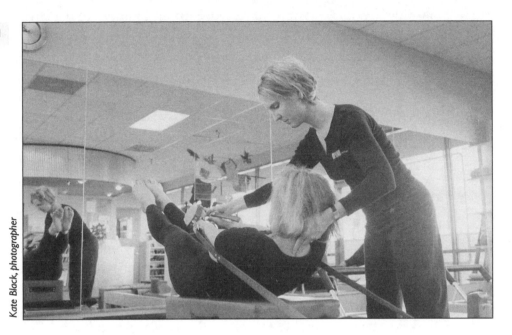

Kate Black, photographer

The Principle of Proper Breathing

Proper breathing guides everything else you do in your Pilates training. To breathe properly during Pilates exercises, you need to fill your lungs completely – expanding them to their greatest capacity – and then empty the lungs of all air. The more deeply you breathe in and the more fully you exhale, the better you will nourish and cleanse your body. Try it right now, and note what a difference it makes in the way you feel.

In Pilates, breathing and movement are closely coordinated. When you read instructions for Pilates movements, you'll see that you're told when to inhale and when to exhale. Follow those directions carefully to get the most from the Pilates exercises.

The Fundamental Goals of Pilates

The fundamental goals of Pilates are uniform development, proper breathing, flexible and decompressed spine and joints, robust circulation and a unity of body/mind/spirit. When you focus your mind to control and coordinate your movements, your body develops more uniformly, and your spine and joints achieve a healthy range of motion, thereby promoting increased circulation and breathing capacity. This, in turn, brings more life-giving oxygen to all your tissues. Pilates achieves these goals through the guiding principles listed earlier in this chapter. The following sections describe each of the Pilates goals in further detail.

Body/Mind/Spirit Balance

By emphasizing the importance of the mind/body connection in attaining physical fitness, Joseph Pilates was marrying critical elements of Eastern and Western philosophies. Physical strength, ability and beauty are central to the Western concept of fitness and good health. Westerners approach health and fitness as a scientific function of maintaining and nurturing the body's muscles, bones and circulatory and digestive systems. Eastern philosophies, on the other hand, place much more importance on the development of mental and spiritual powers in the pursuit of pure health. Eastern teachings, such as Buddhism and yoga, direct followers to seek mental peace and inner harmony if they want to be ultimately fit. Physical conditioning is intertwined with mental and spiritual development, through controlled breathing and meditation. The ancient practice of yoga is extremely popular today, in part due to its strong emphasis on the mind/body fitness connection.

Joseph Pilates based his fitness programme and philosophy on a foundation that straddled both Eastern and Western concepts. Pilates students approach each movement with focus and determination, and they engage body and mind equally in each physical endeavour.

Uniform Development

Pilates isn't a bodybuilder's workout, designed to bulk up your pecs or give you bulging muscles. Pilates is a conditioning programme designed to work the whole body simultaneously and uniformly. Joseph Pilates created his exercises with the intention 'that each muscle may cooperatively and loyally aid in the uniform development of all our muscles. Developing minor muscles naturally helps to strengthen major muscles'. As a result, every muscle is developed in every movement.

> Pilates truly does work to develop longer, stronger muscles – not just bigger ones. Pilates benefits also extend beyond your muscles, to develop stronger, more flexible joints, as well. Regular Pilates practice helps you build a strong, flexible, uniformly well-developed body.

Joseph Pilates believed in the body's natural architectural 'rightness', but he also felt that most people develop ways of standing, sitting and moving that interfere with their body's structural integrity. Pilates designed his exercises and movements to bring people back to this natural state – a state that promotes regeneration instead of degeneration. Uniform development ensures that the body is aligned as it should be, with all joints supported by balanced weight and force.

Proper Breathing

Remember that proper breathing is both a guiding principle and a goal of the Pilates method because it is so essential to good health. Joseph Pilates designed his method with an overriding goal of improving the way the human body is nourished through breathing. The human body needs oxygen, and the lungs are responsible for feeding that oxygen to the body's cells through the bloodstream. When you breathe in, your lungs fill with air and extract oxygen from it; when you breathe out, your lungs push out carbon dioxide and eliminate waste products your body doesn't need. When you breathe properly, you have more stamina, feel more alive and alert, and are better able to concentrate.

Many Pilates exercises involve an action known as 'rolling'. Spine-rolling exercises offer good opportunities for really cleaning out the lungs. According to Pilates, 'It is this very action of rolling and unrolling that cleanses your lungs so effectively by driving out the impure air and forcing in the pure air'. You will learn more about spine rolling later in the book, but here's a short guide to this movement. When you roll your spine in Pilates, you roll one vertebra at a time 'exactly in imitation of a wheel rolling forwards and backwards'. When you roll forwards, your body's action helps push the air out of your lungs; when you roll backwards, your lungs naturally expand to fill again with fresh, pure air.

Joseph Pilates believed the concept of cleansing the lungs by rolling the spine was so important that he created many exercises that incorporate this spinal massaging movement. You perform rolling movements from a lying-down position, a kneeling position, a sitting position, a standing position and even while twisting. In any position, the rolling movement helps intensify your full, complete breathing.

Ready to practise Pilates breathing? Try this exercise:

1. Sit upright in your chair, feet flat on the floor, and place the palms of your hands on either side of your ribcage.
2. Take a deep breath in through your nose, with your lips closed, and expand your ribs outward into your hands as far as they'll go; fill your lungs with air until you feel they can't take in any more.
3. Open your mouth, draw your belly in and up along the front of your spine, and push your palms into your ribcage to squeeze all the air out of your lungs. Deflate your lungs completely, remembering to squeeze every atom of air from them.
4. Repeat steps 2 and 3 up to five times.

Note that when you've emptied your lungs completely, your next inhale happens automatically and is very deep. That's because your lungs were so empty that the more completely you exhale, the more deeply (and easily) you inhale.

Flexible and Decompressed Spine and Joints

Pilates believed long, strong bodies don't just look better – they function better, too. That's why flexibility, decompression and elongation of your body – muscles and joints, including the very important spinal column – –are fundamental goals of the Pilates method of body conditioning.

Your spine is a complex and elegant construction, beautifully designed to bend, twist and provide a strong central support for your body's framework and internal organs. Unfortunately, many people maintain a posture that doesn't support the spine's natural, necessary range of movement, and therefore they limit their spine's strength and capability. If you doubt that most people don't know how to best use and protect their spines, consider that back pain is a leading cause of workplace absences.

In addition to their other benefits, Pilates movements are specifically designed to elongate, strengthen and decompress the spine and joints. This work makes you taller, stronger and better balanced. This tall, upright stance also gives your lungs room to expand, and gives all your organs the space they need to function at peak health and efficiency in your body. Decompressed joints throughout your body give you increased strength, mobility and energy.

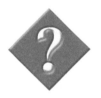

Why do hands and feet get cold and joints ache?
Decompressed joints promote better, more complete circulation. When a joint is no longer tight, imbalanced, torqued or compressed, blood can flow in and around the joint more readily, thereby nourishing the joint tissue and promoting better joint health.

Having a flexible, elongated spine is important for more than just its structural support. Your ribs attach directly to your spine, so if your spine is stiff and hunched you can't breathe deeply and effectively. And if your spine isn't strong, flexible and well-aligned, you place damaging strain on all the other joints and muscles in your body.

Robust Circulation

Your body's circulatory system is its life source, and achieving a strong, healthy circulatory system is a primary goal of the Pilates method. All Pilates exercises and movements increase your heart rate and help boost circulation to speed fresh, oxygenated blood throughout your body.

Pilates breathing is an equally important part of the 'circulation equation'. When you breathe fully and deeply, expanding and contracting your lungs completely with each breath, you help boost the oxygen in your bloodstream. Deep Pilates breathing also helps gets your heart pumping to stimulate the blood's circulation.

In other words, Pilates breathing and movement techniques improve the quality of nourishment in your blood, and they improve your body's delivery system for sending that nourishing blood to the muscles, organs, bones and connective tissues of your body.

'Breathing is the first act of life, and the last. Our very life depends on it... millions and millions... have never learned to master the art of correct breathing. One often wonders how so many millions continue to live as long as they do under this tremendous handicap to longevity. Therefore, above all, learn how to breathe correctly.'

Joseph Pilates, *Return to Life Through Contrology*

CHAPTER 4

Choosing Your Training Location and Instructor

You know what the Pilates method is, how it was developed, and the fundamental principles and goals of Pilates body conditioning. Now it's time to decide how you intend to study this method – and you have many options. All around the world, Pilates facilities are teaching tens of thousands of students the techniques, philosophies and exercises of the Pilates method, but how do you find the right one for you?

Studying in a Pilates Facility

Why is studying in a professional environment under an instructor's guidance so important? First, a teacher's trained and watchful eye can ensure that you develop only good habits as you learn the Pilates method of body conditioning. In addition, working in a professional environment is a stimulating and educational experience. You learn by observing other people working out – seeing and hearing the teachers and other students in the process of learning and practising Pilates.

It's highly recommended that you get your doctor's approval before you start any fitness programme, and that includes Pilates. If your doctor is unfamiliar with Pilates, take this book along with you to your next appointment, so your doctor can get a quick, concise outline of the programme.

Watching and listening as the instructor guides another student through a Pilates movement will give you insights and inspirations that help improve your own technique. A correction given to another client might be just the thing to turn on that proverbial light bulb for you. And this instructional environment isn't just helpful for beginners, either; no matter how advanced your Pilates training and experience might be, you'll always find that an instructor's guidance is valuable. Your Pilates workouts will change your body; and your instructor will make sure your Pilates exercises continue to benefit your development.

Choosing a Pilates Place

Depending upon where you live, you may have many different types of Pilates facilities to choose from. Your personal preferences and lifestyle might determine what environment works best for you.

Pilates studios are facilities that are devoted primarily to the instruction of Pilates and little else. Because these businesses focus solely on Pilates, they can tailor your Pilates sessions to your special fitness or rehabilitation needs. A good studio has a number of teachers to choose from, and a full complement of all the Pilates equipment. A fully equipped and staffed studio can offer a large range of appointment and class times, and many types of sessions, including private, small groups and slightly larger classes. Studios are typically set up on a pay-by-session or -class basis, not by membership. An initial one-to-one session is recommended before facing a class or studio environment, and there may be a small reduction if you book a number of sessions at a time.

Health clubs and recreation centres offer Pilates along with many other fitness activities, such as yoga and aerobics. Such clubs usually require a membership, and for that fee, most clubs provide additional services, including swimming pools, squash courts, aerobic equipment and saunas. Pilates classes at these centres typically stress mat work, because they rarely have equipment, and the mat-work classes can be quite large and very mixed in level, which may not address your needs. Many clubs and recreation centres consider Pilates to be an extra and charge an added fee, so ask for details.

Large Pilates mat-work classes don't allow instructors to spend much time with individual students. Especially if you're seeking Pilates for physical rehabilitation of an injury or chronic illness, one of these large group classes is not the answer for you.

Medical offices, such as those under the direction of chiropractors and physical therapists, often offer Pilates sessions. In these settings, the focus is on rehabilitation, not fitness. These offices may be small and intimate, and offer only one-on-one instruction. Pilates may be covered by your health or car insurance (in case of injuries due to car accidents), and medical staff are trained in understanding insurance billing procedures.

Due to their size, however, many medical offices use only a few selected pieces of Pilates equipment and may have only one or two Pilates instructors. Although you may be limited in your choice of instructors or time slots, you may receive professional medical guidance along with your Pilates instruction at a medical office – depending on the nature of your injury or rehabilitation needs, that guidance may be a useful benefit.

Dance schools sometimes offer Pilates instruction as well. Dancers were among the first to discover Pilates, and the dance community continues to understand and depend on its physical rehabilitation and conditioning benefits. Many dance schools offer private instruction or classes; others know of someone who teaches Pilates locally. If you're having difficulty finding a Pilates instructor, try calling your local dance school. They may know your best and closest source for Pilates training.

Home studios are another option for studying the Pilates method of body conditioning. Many individual instructors set up shop in a back room or basement. Although this is not always the case, these small studios may have limited equipment and space; and more than likely, the owner is the only instructor. Home studios are intimate, personal, quiet and can be informal (you might have to walk through the kitchen and share the toilet with the family).

Points to Consider

You can decide which Pilates environment best suits your needs, based on convenience, price, location and personal preference. As with any fitness facility or programme, your perfect Pilates place will need to meet a number of requirements. Think about these:

· **Location.** Will you be going to your Pilates session from home, work or both? How far is too far to discourage regular attendance? Is the facility near other important destinations? Can you combine your Pilates with essential errands such as shopping or stopping at the dry cleaners? Don't discount the importance of convenience. No matter how much you want to be committed to your Pilates programme, if getting to your session takes too much time, you'll be prone to skipping it – and that's no good for you or your Pilates programme.

· **Cost.** Pilates isn't the lowest-cost fitness programme out there, but it's worth every penny. That said, high price doesn't always mean best quality. Some of the best facilities have very reasonable price, and some of the worst overcharge. Don't choose a facility by finding the one that provides the cheapest sessions in your area, but make sure you're realistic in determining how much you can afford to spend on your

Pilates programme. 'It's too expensive' can become a reason to drop out. Ask for a full schedule of all costs – membership fees, individual sessions, package deals, equipment use, parking and so on.

· **Support staff.** In addition to your instructor, are support personnel available to help you? Can you easily contact someone to change appointments or discuss your billing? Are the people helpful, friendly and willing to assist you when necessary? Many facilities are too small to offer support staff, so the teacher may also handle reception, class scheduling, cleaning and so on. Is that all right with you?

· **Class structure.** If you intend to study in group classes, find out how those classes are organized. Will you be able to work with a group of others who share your fitness/experience level? If you're just starting your Pilates training, you don't want to be the lone beginner in a class of advanced students; as you advance, you don't want to be hindered by newcomers. Ask about class sizes, too; you can get lost in classes of more than ten students.

· **Other programmes and services.** Does the facility offer other health and fitness programmes, such as physical therapy, aerobics, massage, on-site snack bar or nutritional counselling? How about on-site child care? Are these services something you're interested in?

Be aware of the cost of quitting. If you sign up for a six-month Pilates training programme, do you have to pay the entire fee in advance? What happens if you have to drop out of the programme after two months? Make sure you find out the policy on refunds, and read any contracts carefully before signing.

Shop around, visit the various Pilates facilities and ask if you can observe group classes and private sessions. Do the clients look as if they're having a good time? Is the teacher focused on instruction, or is he or she answering the telephone, eating and chatting about everything but Pilates? Check out the condition of the equipment and the cleanliness of the changing rooms. Get a feel for the atmosphere. Is it bright and inviting, or more like a fitness dungeon? How does it sound? Is it noisy, with lots of loud music and television chatter, or is it relatively quiet? You can't concentrate on your movements and body response when you're surrounded by bedlam. At the same time, instructors should be actively engaged with students and the atmosphere should feel warm and inviting, not stern and severe.

There are a number of websites designed to help you find a local Pilates instructor, in addition to looking in the Yellow Pages for your area. Check Appendix A for these.

As you've learned when you work in a full Pilates facility, you have the opportunity to participate in private sessions, mat work and equipment classes. We recommend you take advantage of all these types of Pilates sessions. Unlike some other forms of fitness, Pilates is designed to be done every day. With all these options open to you, you can devise a programme that is interesting, variable, affordable, fun, challenging and rewarding to your mind and body.

Your First Evaluation Session

Ideally, your very first session will be a personal one-to-one evaluation of you and your body. That way, your Pilates instructor can help ensure that your programme will be able to meet your needs and goals. Instructor attention and assistance are critical for getting the most from your Pilates programme.

An evaluation session includes a brief discussion of your present physical condition, your medical history as it applies to your Pilates training, and your fitness needs and goals. Your first session should also include a workout, during which your instructor can learn more about your body and the way it moves. This knowledge will help the instructor devise a good Pilates programme for you. The result of your first session should be that you leave feeling rejuvenated, taller and excited about your newfound opportunity to 'return to life'.

Arrive for your first session early enough to get acquainted with the facility and its amenities. After you've settled in, you will be asked to fill out a questionnaire to provide information regarding your health, medical history, lifestyle, fitness goals, rehabilitation needs and so on. Your instructor will give you a chance to ask questions, express concerns and otherwise make yourself feel comfortable and acquainted with the instructor and the facility. Your instructor will also take this opportunity to assess your body posture, condition and alignment, and ask any questions necessary to help understand how to begin teaching you.

Benefiting from Pilates Group Sessions

If your chosen facility doesn't offer private sessions or individual introductory evaluation sessions, you will probably use an introductory group session to become familiar with the Pilates method and their way of teaching it; by definition, however, this type of session can't offer a personal evaluation of your specific needs and goals.

A good Pilates facility limits class size to enable instructors to spend adequate amounts of time with everyone. Eight to ten people is a good size for a group that does mat work, and equipment classes should be made up of no more than six students. Larger classes limit the amount of individual attention you receive – and the quality of your workout.

A good Pilates instructor should be capable of teaching the entire group while also giving some individual guidance to students as necessary. The instructor is able to help each person get the most from the class and keep the class moving through the Pilates exercises with rhythm and flow.

What to Expect in Group Sessions

Classes are a step toward making Pilates your own. Because an instructor is giving you less personal attention than in a private session, you become responsible for some of your own instruction and guidance. With less input from an outside source, your mind is freed to focus more on your internal voice and to experience your teacher's input in new ways. This focus allows you to deepen your personal understanding of the Pilates movements and exercises. In addition, you can use this as an opportunity to recall and put into use past corrections and directions you've received in your Pilates instruction.

Group sessions offer you an opportunity to develop your awareness and concentration. Because you can't rely solely on the teacher in this situation, you prepare yourself to do your homework better. Equally important, the group energy and supportiveness of your classmates can inspire you to new heights, to gain new capabilities that you didn't even know were possible.

Many Pilates instructors regularly study in group classes in order to get a fresh perspective on the Pilates method and learn something more about the way they, themselves, move. This gives them the opportunity to hear the types of questions asked and interactions the students have with another instructor, which in turn improves their own teaching skills.

Most Pilates group sessions last for approximately one hour, and cost anywhere from £7 (for a large mat class in a recreation centre) to £20 per session (for an equipment session with two or three students); the average price for a one-to-one session is £40.

Costs vary depending upon the facility, location, the type and size of classes and so on. Some facilities offer the options of independent workout time, and many offer package deals, as well as discounts for bulk bookings. Be sure to ask for a fee schedule.

Taking Pilates Mat-Work Classes

Mat-work classes (see FIGURE 4-1) vary with each facility and instructor; most include 20 students or fewer, and last from one to one-and-a-half hours. Because the instructor doesn't have to monitor the use of the equipment, mat-work classes require somewhat less intensive supervision and instruction than students require in equipment classes. For this reason, mat classes may include more students than equipment classes.

In general, mat-work classes are less expensive than equipment classes; expect to pay £7 to £10 per session. Your facility and instructor can give you full details.

FIGURE 4-1

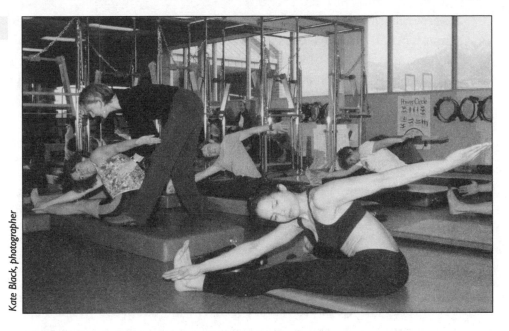

Kate Black, photographer

Official Pilates mats are made of high-density foam and are equipped with a foot strap and weighted bar. Mat-work classes may include other equipment, such as stretch bands, balls and foam rollers, weights and Magic Circles. You and your fellow students work through the same sets of exercises simultaneously, with the instructor moving among you and assisting as necessary. Some studios require you to sign up for mat-work classes, while other facilities let you drop in. Make sure to ask.

Some Pilates facilities have a session cancellation policy that holds you responsible for paying for unattended sessions unless you offer a 24-hour notice that you'll be unable to attend. That gives the instructor an opportunity to fill your slot and sets a standard of mutual respect.

Mat classes can provide an aerobic workout of varying intensity, depending on your fitness and skill level, and your facility's approach. These classes can be a lot of fun; students develop a strong sense of camaraderie and offer each other mutual support and encouragement.

Remember that Joe Pilates designed his equipment work to facilitate the mat work. If you have the Pilates equipment available to you, take advantage of it, but always balance your Pilates programme with both kinds of sessions. That's the best way to get the most benefit from Pilates.

Studying in Pilates Equipment Classes

When you study in a Pilates equipment class, your instructor will introduce you to the features of each piece of equipment and show you the proper way to use it (you get a full description of all of the most important pieces of Pilates equipment in Chapter 6). Classes may be offered with Universal Reformers and Trapeze Table/Pole Systems, as well as Chairs, Barrels and Magic Circles.

Never attempt to use Pilates equipment without proper training and supervision! Pilates equipment offers multiple health and fitness benefits, but each piece has unique and important safety requirements. Don't underestimate the necessity for proper training in the use of each piece.

Although you need an instructor's training to use Pilates equipment safely and effectively, don't be put off by this fact or by the imposing appearance of some pieces. The amazing results you can achieve from using the Pilates equipment are worth far more than the time and attention you invest in the learning experience. A good instructor will walk you through the process and ensure that your equipment experience is safe, productive – and fun!

Pilates equipment uses straps, springs and pulleys to offer variable resistance as you perform Pilates movements. These pieces help you maintain the proper position during your exercises and guide your body's movement, so you can do more and get better, quicker results than you can achieve on your own (see FIGURE 4-2).

Most equipment classes are smaller than mat classes. Expect to study with ten or fewer fellow students – the number varies according to the facility's size and equipment availability. Smaller is better for equipment group classes, with six students being the ideal maximum size. Because equipment classes require more management and supervision, they cost a bit more than mat-work classes; expect to pay between £15 and £30 for a small group equipment session of two to eight people.

FIGURE 4-2

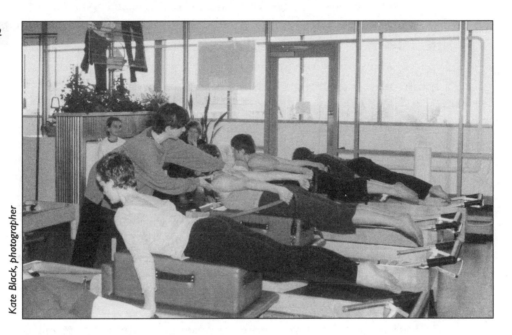

Kate Black, photographer

Working in Private Pilates Sessions

Uniform development is the hallmark of the Pilates method. A certified instructor's trained eye, focused directly and solely on your form and technique and your body's individual needs, will help you progress more quickly. An instructor can spot subtle, inefficient movement patterns and give you very personal, specific instructions to address these problems.

Try to make personal instruction a part of your programme whenever you can, no matter how advanced and independent you become in your Pilates training. Frequent or infrequent private sessions serve as 'clean-ups' to ensure that you're continuing to get the most from your Pilates programme.

Individual sessions are especially helpful if you have an injury or trying to break long-established movement patterns that are inefficient or detrimental to your posture, joints and overall health. Nothing works better for your body's development than individual Pilates sessions.

Private sessions offer benefits beyond the instructor's undivided attention. Because you're working individually, private sessions usually offer more flexibility in scheduling. And, knowing that an instructor is expecting to work with you alone can spur you on to keep your appointment, rather than missing it because 'no one will notice'.

What to Expect from a Private Session

If you're studying Pilates in private sessions only, plan to schedule one from once to three times a week, depending on your time, needs and financial situation. However, if you're working out at home and in group classes as well, you might need to meet for a private session less frequently. Your private sessions will last approximately an hour. The cost of private sessions varies dramatically; you can expect to pay between £30 and £60 per session.

Don't be surprised if your instructor uses his or her hands to move you into the correct positions or guide you through the Pilates movements (see FIGURE 4-3). Let your instructor know what kind of hands-on guidance works best for you.

It is highly recommended that you begin your Pilates studies with a few weeks of private sessions before moving into group sessions. You can always benefit from doing Pilates in a group – at any level of accomplishment – but the benefits of private instruction are worth every penny. Talk with your instructor to decide what combination of group and private sessions will work best for you. You don't need to worry about overdoing it; you can do Pilates every day, because the system offers so many exercise and movement options, and it doesn't focus on any particular set of muscles.

FIGURE 4-3

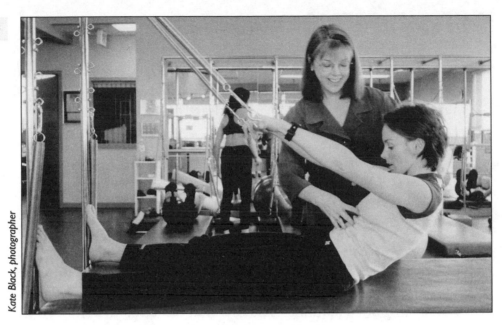

Kate Black, photographer

What Are Your Instructor's Qualifications?

Unfortunately, lots of people who claim they teach the methods of Joseph Pilates aren't really teaching those methods at all, and many facilities that claim to offer Pilates training don't have a clear sense of what the Pilates method really is. If you want to study and practise Pilates – the method of body conditioning as envisioned and created by Joseph Pilates himself – you should look for a highly qualified, preferably certified instructor and a reputable facility.

When a facility or instructor claims to offer the Pilates method of body conditioning, as created by Joseph Pilates, find out where or with whom the instructor received Pilates training or certification, what that training programme entailed and how long it lasted. Ask the instructor what other influences he or she draws from. And remember, you learn a lot about Joseph Pilates's methods in this book; use the information here to help separate the Pilates pretenders from the real thing.

What Does Pilates Certification Mean?

If a Pilates instructor is certified, does that mean you can relax and start training? Not exactly. Certification programmes vary in quality, content and value. That instructor's certification may be gold standard, or it might not be worth the paper it's printed on.

For the authoritative source on Pilates certification programmes, contact the Pilates Method Alliance; you can visit the website at www.pilatesmethodalliance.org.

Because there's been a high demand for certified Pilates instructors over the past few years, a number of 'fast-through'–type certification programmes have sprung up to answer the call. These programmes focus on getting out a minimum amount of information in a short time, trying to meet the demand of health clubs and so on (in fact, after reading this book you may know more than some of these instructors). In some of these programmes, applicants pay a fee, attend a weekend-long session of instructor training and emerge on Monday morning with certification in hand. In this case, the problem isn't whether the instructors are getting what they paid for; the problem is that future students will get just what these instructors have paid for – and that isn't much.

A reputable Pilates certification programme requires a long-term commitment to a rigorous training routine that involves a variety of components, including an advanced understanding and ability with the techniques of Pilates, a basic understanding of anatomy, training in using and instructing others in Pilates equipment exercises, a specific number of hours of formal lecture, apprenticeship study, personal training and an in-depth certification examination process. Most reputable training programmes require months and even years of study. In addition, most also require annual recertification study. In other words, becoming a truly qualified and certified Pilates instructor requires a long-term professional commitment (see Chapter 21 for more information).

Finding the Right Instructor for You

Taking lessons with a highly trained Pilates instructor is the best way to ensure successful progress in your Pilates programme. In many parts of the country, you won't have much trouble locating a Pilates instructor. In fact, this book includes a list of Pilates training associations that advertise their certified instructors on their websites in Appendix A, along with some additional resources for finding facilities in your area. So if you have a number of reputable Pilates instructors to choose from, how do you choose?

Everyone who teaches Pilates is unique and brings his or her own sets of strengths and weaknesses to the studio or classroom. But in general, here are some traits to look for in a good Pilates instructor. If you're observing instructors in action, check this list to see how they measure up on the traits that matter most to you. A good Pilates instructor is:

· Adept in the full repertoire of all the Pilates exercises, at all levels and on all equipment.
· A long-term and ongoing practitioner and student of Pilates.
· Able to verify completion of training or certification in Pilates.
· Taking continuing education courses to remain fresh and invigorated in his/her own teaching.
· Knowledgeable about basic anatomy.
· Able to demonstrate a strong background in Pilates history and philosophy.
· A good example of what Pilates can do for the body.
· A professional who maintains professional boundaries (in other words, avoids bringing personal issues and inappropriate comments or advances into the lesson).
· Capable of helping clients progress safely and effectively through the advancing levels of Pilates.
· Motivating, encouraging and inspiring to clients.

In addition, a good Pilates instructor should be well versed in: safety; hands-on and modification techniques; all transitions between exercises; and the major benefits and skills derived from each exercise.

As you observe the instructor in action, look for some of the skills any good teacher exhibits. The instructor should speak clearly, concisely and authoritatively, without being arrogant or demeaning. Good instructors are in constant communication with their students, using their voices, hands and eyes to give and receive information. After the session, students of a good Pilates teacher should leave feeling taller and rejuvenated, more knowledgeable about their bodies and Pilates, and calm and connected in body, mind and spirit.

It's an Important Decision

Pilates is an exact – and exacting – method, and its students need and deserve a well-educated instructor, someone who's been a long-time student of Pilates and who experienced the challenges and growth of an extensive, intensive certification process; someone who's developed the rich understanding that accompanies the evolution of knowledge and skill. Your Pilates programme will require a real commitment on your part; make sure you find someone with whom you feel comfortable in making that commitment, so you can be partners in your progress.

CHAPTER 5

Doing Your Pilates Homework

Working out in a Pilates facility with the help and guidance of a well-trained, certified instructor is the best way to go, but Pilates work at home is also strongly recommended. This book describes a number of effective home workout techniques and exercises – but they're not meant to replace studying in a professional environment.

Practising Pilates at Home

Joseph Pilates intended every student to do some Pilates work at home. This book offers step-by-step techniques for many Pilates movements and exercises. If you follow those instructions carefully, you can achieve a safe, healthy and beneficial Pilates workout in any space large enough to lie down in and spread out your arms and legs.

Finding a Good Workout Space

You can put together your own home studio environment without a lot of fuss or expense. Here are some simple recommendations:

· Find a space large enough for a mat, where you feel comfortable lying down, standing up, kicking your legs and stretching your arms, without banging into walls, obstacles, furniture and so on.
· Have plenty of clean, fresh air available to you as you deep-breathe your way through your Pilates workout. A well-ventilated room that isn't draughty and has an even temperature is ideal.
· Work out away from the phone, doorbell and other distractions, and don't go for the background music you might have used in other types of workouts; let your body and your breath set the rhythm and tempo for your workout.

Getting Together Your Equipment

You don't need an arsenal of equipment to enjoy an effective, productive session of Pilates at home. As you become more experienced in Pilates, you may choose to purchase some official Pilates equipment, but in the beginning, your home Pilates studio can be very simply equipped (see FIGURE 5-1).

· Get a good workout mat that is firm yet provides good cushioning for your spine and pelvic bones. A yoga mat is too thin for most people, and your bed won't provide the stability and support you need for mat-work exercises. You can purchase a Pilates mat, or improvise one by using a high-density foam camping pad. Make sure that it provides a thick cushion between your spine, pelvis and floor, and that it isn't slippery. (You learn more about the construction of a Pilates mat in Chapter 6; Appendix B lists sources for purchasing Pilates mats.)

· If you have a large mirror, position it so you can see yourself during your Pilates exercises. You can visually check the position of your pelvis, arms, legs and neck by comparing them to the instructions and photos in this book. Again, you need to be very precise in performing your Pilates exercises and movements; a mirror will give you a visual check on that precision.

FIGURE 5-1

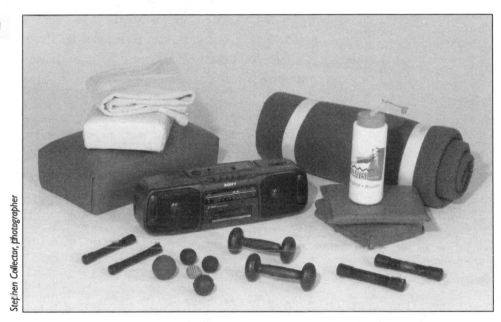

Stephen Collector, photographer

· It can be helpful to audiotape or videotape one of your Pilates sessions in which a teacher is giving you instruction. You can follow the recording when you're working out at home. Check that your instructor is happy for you to do this.

· Although not essential, many people like to use light weights (no more than 1.5kg/3lb) in some Pilates exercises and movements. Tins of soup make excellent, low-cost Pilates weights! If you choose to use weights, have them nearby during your workout, so you don't interrupt the flow of your session.

· Many people find that small pillows provide a necessary positioning boost when doing Pilates mat-work exercises. As you learn the Pilates exercise techniques in Chapters 8–19, you may discover that this kind of support works well for you, too. Again, have them nearby so you needn't stop and search for them during your workout.

· An assortment of small balls of different sizes, ranging from squash balls to children's play balls can come in handy as well. Ask your instructor for guidance on how to use these.

· Always have a water bottle nearby during your workout. You'll frequently want to rehydrate your system, and the closer your water source, the sooner you can resume your workout.

· Keep this book nearby as well. You can refer to it in order to review forgotten details, to help you better understand your evolving capabilities and to inspire you to further challenges.

Always 'listen' to your body during your Pilates workout, and don't push yourself to do anything that's painful or uncomfortable. In the studio, your instructor may encourage you to attempt challenging movements. But when you work alone, it's particularly important to avoid any position or movement that feels beyond your capabilities.

Your Pilates Partner

When you work out in a Pilates facility, the instructor will walk you through the steps of each Pilates exercise or movement, and help you assume the right positions, movements and pace for your specific needs. When you're on your own, you need some other strategies for learning and performing the Pilates exercises.

If possible, arrange for a friend or workout partner to run through the first few home sessions with you. Your partner can read the exercise steps from this book, check your position/technique against the descriptions in this book and help you perform the exercises more precisely.

If you return the favour by helping your partner work through the exercises, you get another learning boost in return. As your partner performs the movements, keep a careful watch on his or her body for signs of strain or improper technique. Watching someone else do the exercises while you read the instructions is a good way to learn the Pilates essentials when you don't have the aid of a certified instructor. In addition, you may inspire a new fan of Pilates who could become your workout partner. Working out can be more fun with a partner, and you may be more likely to stay committed to your Pilates workouts when you know another person is counting on you.

However, *you* can be your own partner. Write exercise steps and important guidelines, reminders and other tips, on poster-size paper and tape them on a nearby wall (or even the ceiling!). Alternatively, read the exercise steps from this book into a cassette recorder, then play back the tape as you work through the exercises. You may need to remake and refine this recording as you progress in your own abilities and as you determine what verbal cues and reminders work best for you.

Your Home Workout Schedule

Joseph Pilates had several words of advice to offer those just beginning their Pilates study at home. First, he counselled that it's extremely important that you practise every day – even if in the beginning you practise for only ten minutes at a time. After a week or so, you may find yourself able to extend your workout times to 20 minutes, 30 minutes or more. Pilates believed that anyone's concentration will falter after about 45 minutes or so, so don't overextend yourself. The Pilates method is designed to work most effectively when done frequently – even every day – for short periods of time.

What to Wear

Don't laugh – you might be surprised to know how many students are confused about just what to wear to a Pilates workout. In *Return to Life Through Contrology*, Joseph Pilates recommended that people wear as little as possible when exercising; Pilates himself is shown wearing a bathing suit in nearly every photograph ever taken of him doing his exercises or helping others in the Pilates's studio.

Pilates students wear no shoes, because foot movement and placement are critical in the Pilates method. If you're working out in a Pilates facility, you might be required to wear clean socks or gymnastic-type slippers for sanitary reasons. Remember, you can always ask your instructor for specific ideas regarding the right workout wear for your programme.

Does that mean you have to wear a Speedo or bikini to get Pilates-fit? Not at all. In fact, most Pilates students wear leotards, leggings, shorts, bike shorts, tank tops, T-shirts, light sweatsuits or similar workout wear. Heavy or bulky sweatsuits aren't good Pilates choices, however. You need to be able to see your body, its muscles and movements during each Pilates exercise. Don't wear belts or any clothing that will bunch up or create lumps under your body or constrict movement when you work out; you don't want to hurt yourself when you roll up on your spine or press your pelvis into the mat. Sports bras are a good idea for women, and men should wear some sort of athletic support (and avoid running shorts that are loose around the legs). Tie your hair back and remove all jewellery.

Decide What Works Best for You

All the exercise instructions in this book include guidelines on the number of repetitions of any one exercise to be performed in any one session. Be certain to always follow these recommendations. Remember, in Pilates you don't advance by crunching out more reps – you advance by learning to perform each movement and exercise with awareness, breathing, concentration, centring, precise control, flowing movement and oppositional energy.

Finally, put together the schedule that works best for you. You can work out in the morning, afternoon or evening – whatever time suits you best. Here are some additional guidelines to remember in constructing your schedule:

- Don't work out immediately after you've eaten; your body is busy digesting its food, so let your Pilates workout wait until it can hold all your body's energy and attention. (How can you pull in your stomach when it's full, anyway?)
- If you're suffering from a cold, flu or other illness, don't push yourself through a Pilates workout. Pilates is a refreshing, invigorating exercise, but it also demands physical and mental stamina!

If you're ill, you won't be able to perform well, and you'll use up energy that can best be put to work towards your recovery. On the other hand, a good workout, appropriately adjusted for your state of health, can flush your system clear of toxins by creating an 'internal shower'. Take it easy, don't push yourself and remember your water bottle!

Common Sense

You've read a number of cautions throughout this book, but it's appropriate to repeat a few of them here. Pilates is a serious fitness programme, so you need to approach it seriously. Keep these warnings and points of advice in mind when you begin your Pilates study:

- Follow your doctor's instructions for any restrictions on your movements or activities (remember, you need to discuss the programme with your doctor before you begin, and get approval).
- Listen to your body. Any time something hurts or feels uncomfortable, stop the movement, get out of the position and tell your instructor. Minor discomfort or exertion is natural, but Pilates isn't a no-pain-no-gain type of exercise. You shouldn't have to strain excessively or tolerate pain during your session.
- Don't overextend. If a stretch or movement feels uncomfortable, try shortening the length a bit. As your body becomes more 'Pilates-ized', you'll be able to safely and comfortably extend your stretch, so don't be a hero and strain your muscles and joints by asking too much too soon.

· If an injury has kept you from your Pilates practice, have a discussion with your instructor before resuming your workouts, so you can coordinate your continued Pilates training with your doctor or rehabilitation specialist.

All Systems Go!

With the information you've received up to this point in the book, you're now prepared to begin a safe, effective and energizing programme in the Pilates method of body conditioning. In later chapters, you'll learn some of the Pilates mat work, along with helpful modifications to tailor those movements to your abilities and fitness goals. Don't forget the helpful information offered in the preceding chapters of this book, and return to these chapters for a refresher whenever you feel the need. There's a lot to know about Pilates; take time to learn as much as you can. The rewards are never-ending, ever-evolving and fabulously life-enhancing.

'Patience and Persistence are vital qualities in the ultimate successful accomplishment of any worthwhile endeavour.'

Joseph Pilates, *Return to Life Through Contrology*

CHAPTER 6

Pilates Equipment

Pilates is a system of exercise that combines mat-work and equipment exercises. This chapter offers you an introduction to the equipment you will likely encounter in a Pilates studio. (Most of the Pilates equipment shown in this chapter is manufactured by Peak Body Systems, of Boulder, Colorado, USA.)

The Universal Reformer

The Universal Reformer is the most widely known piece of Pilates equipment and is an amazingly versatile apparatus. The Universal Reformer's unique combination of springs, pulleys, straps and sliding carriage make it an incredibly valuable and useful piece of equipment. Its adjustability enables the Reformer to address a wide range of physical capabilities, disabilities and fitness goals with refined, sophisticated solutions. Joseph Pilates created nearly 100 exercises on the Reformer – more exercises than he designed for any other piece of Pilates equipment.

How the Universal Reformer Works

The Reformer, shown in FIGURE 6-1, consists of a wooden or metal rectangular frame, approximately 2.3m (7ft) long and 61cm (2ft) wide, resting about 40cm (16in) above the floor on four legs – early versions of this piece actually had claw feet! Interior metal tracks run the length of the frame, providing guidance for a wheeled and padded carriage that attaches to the frame with springs at one end and a handle-and-strap pulley system at the other.

FIGURE 6-1

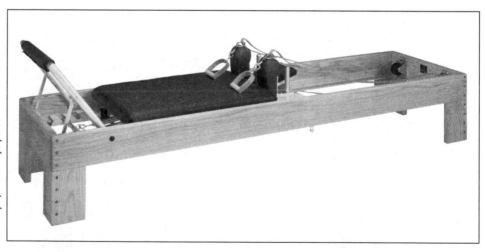

Courtesy of Peak Body Systems

The carriage has a headrest and shoulder blocks, and some have handgrips. One end of the Reformer frame is equipped with a foot bar and strap, and a series of gears that allow users to adjust the distance between the shoulder blocks and foot bar to accommodate different movements and body types.

> Several accessories are available for the Reformer, including additional straps, support blocks, strap extensions and so on. One post-Pilates addition is the Jumpboard – a piece now considered standard with most Reformer models. Pilates master instructor Romana Kryzanowska felt that Joe would have approved of this addition to his classic machine.

On the Reformer, the student lies, sits, kneels and stands in every conceivable position as he or she stretches and extends the body completely – enabling access to a full range of movements and, therefore, developing all of the body's muscles simultaneously. Sometimes the student's hands are on the foot bar, sometimes they hold flexible straps or balance on top of the shoulder blocks; or the student's feet can assume any of these positions. In all positions, the spine arches, twists and flexes as the carriage on which the student's body is positioned moves back and forth.

The Reformer (like most Pilates equipment) differs from traditional fitness equipment in very fundamental ways. Rather than using an isolated set of muscles to move an external force, such as a barbell or stack of weights, you use your Powerhouse to lift and pull your body's weight along with the Reformer's spring-loaded carriage. This action automatically centres you, developing balance, coordination and body/space awareness as it strengthens and stretches your entire body, not just any one isolated set of muscles.

The Reformer Exercises

When Joseph Pilates developed a series of exercises especially for the Universal Reformer, he intended them to be performed in a specific sequence and manner that results in a series of nearly constant, flowing movements. You inhale, recline fluidly onto the Reformer and begin a 30- to 60-minute non-stop workout that finishes as you exhale and return to a standing position. Each exercise prepares your body and mind for the next one – warming your muscles, awakening your mind and body, stimulating your organs, coordinating your breathing and training your muscles to 'fire' in the correct sequence to give you the maximum fitness benefit from the exercise movements.

Universal Reformer Modifications

As with all of his equipment, Joseph Pilates continually experimented and advanced his theories and designs for the Reformer. As a result, he built many versions of the Reformer during his lifetime. Since his death, the Reformer has become the most adapted piece of equipment in the Pilates studio.

Many changes to the original Reformer design have benefited neither the client nor the method; the meddlers frequently had little understanding of Pilates' original vision. Differences in dimensions, for instance, alter certain exercises dramatically enough to make them less valuable, sometimes impossible and, in the worst cases, even dangerous. Further complicating matters, some instructors and Pilates facilities teach only the Reformer exercises – offering instruction in no other part of the Pilates method.

Limiting instruction in this way completely abandons Joseph Pilates's original fitness system concept and practice – of which the Reformer was only one (very important) part. Each piece of equipment, including the mat, supports and augments the others. Pilates never allowed anyone to work on only one part of his or her body or on only one machine; everyone was expected to work through a complete routine on the mat and machines, no matter what problem originally brought them to the studio. When choosing a teacher or facility, make sure the equipment is manufactured by a reputable source and that the instruction covers a full range of Pilates exercises and equipment. In other words, make sure your Pilates experience is complete.

Trapeze Table

The Pilates Trapeze Table comes loaded with everything you could want in an exercise apparatus. The Trapeze Table is another direct descendant of that early Pilates experiment in fitness equipment invention back in the World War I internment camp.

FIGURE 6-2

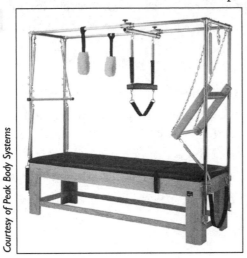

Courtesy of Peak Body Systems

The Trapeze Table consists of a rectangular upholstered platform with metal poles at each corner; the corner poles are connected together at the top by a frame canopy (see FIGURE 6-2). At one end of the Trapeze Table is a swinging bar called the Push Through Bar, which attaches with springs to either the platform or the poles. On the other end, a wooden bar called the Roll Down Bar hangs from the Arm Springs, which are attached to the canopy frame. A set of heavier springs, called the Leg Springs, attach to a series of eye hooks located at varying heights along the support poles. A padded Breathing or Trapeze Bar is connected by springs to a sliding pole on the canopy. A variety of cloth and fleece straps are attached to various places on the Trapeze Table's canopy and platform.

The height of the Trapeze Table platform helps instructors support and assist students as they move through the exercises. The Trapeze Table's straps and bars also work towards this effort, and combine to make the Trapeze Table a perfect tool for injury rehabilitation.

Joseph Pilates created more than 80 exercises for this versatile piece of equipment. Unlike the Reformer exercises, students needn't do all the Trapeze Table exercises in any specific order. The Trapeze Table exercises are designed to correct particular imbalances, and to help students move more quickly towards a uniformly developed body. Like the Reformer, the Trapeze Table exercises build leg strength, upper body power, spinal mobility and stability, always with a strong focus on core or Powerhouse strength.

Pilates allowed his students to name many exercises and pieces of equipment, so it's not uncommon to run across several names for the same item. The Trapeze Table for example, is also referred to as the Trap, or Therapy Table or the Cadillac.

The direct way in which the student's body interacts with the Trapeze Table's springs concentrates the power and effect of each assisted movement specifically in the area of the body the student needs to strengthen or retrain. The Trapeze Table's upper canopy, springs and straps provide for movement possibilities that enable you to engage in exercises ranging from the most gentle to the most extreme – depending upon your needs and abilities.

The Wall Unit or Pole System

FIGURE 6-3

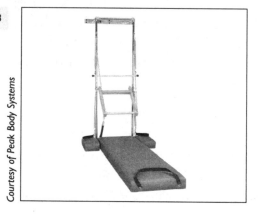

Courtesy of Peak Body Systems

The Wall Unit or Pole System (see FIGURE 6-3) is an adaptation of the Trapeze Table for small spaces, low ceilings or group classes. These smaller pieces of equipment are appropriate for most of the Trapeze Table exercises, with the exception of those that use the upper parallel bars or the canopy frame.

The Chairs

In the Pilates system there are two types of 'chairs': the Low or Wunda Chair, and the High Chair. The main difference between the two types is that the High Chair has a back and two handles that rise on either side of the seat (some Low Chair models also incorporate these handles). Some manufacturers build a Low/High Chair combination unit with a removable back section and handles (see FIGURE 6-4).

FIGURE 6-4

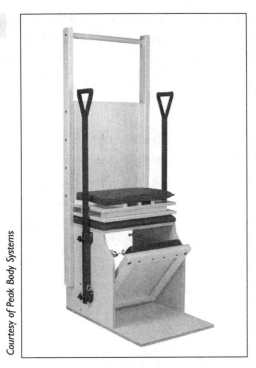

The Chair essentially is a two-sided box with a padded seat. Underneath the seat, a foot pedal attached to the chair with two or four springs provides adjustable tension. Over the years, Pilates constantly revised the Chair, so a number of variations exist, including one with a split foot pedal.

Pilates created the Low Chair (see FIGURE 6-5) for working out at home – as an everyday piece of furniture that doubled as an incredibly versatile exercise apparatus (the Chair could be used as either an occasional table or an armchair – a bonus for small city flats and apartments).

Pictures show Joseph Pilates performing approximately 50 exercises on this multi-purpose apparatus. You can sit, kneel, lie or stand on, in front of or behind the Chair, facing towards or away from it – even sideways – as you move the spring-loaded bar. The Chair's unique and versatile design enables everyone to get amazing results – from the most injured client who uses it to rehabilitate, to the most advanced students challenging themselves with push-ups, backbends and headstands.

FIGURE 6-5

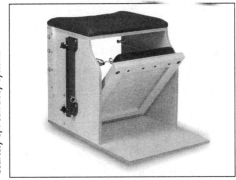

When you add the back piece and the handles, creating a High Chair, the equipment provides even more support and guidance for the body; a handful of exercises are designed specifically for the High Chair. The back piece supports your back during seated exercises, and helps guide your knee through standing exercises. The handles, in conjunction with the spring-loaded foot paddle, enable you to adjust the level of support and resistance as you progressively strengthen your upper body in such Pilates exercises as the Triceps Dips.

What kind of injuries can you rehabilitate with the Chairs?
The Low Chair is particularly effective in working with asymmetrical problems such as knee injury and scoliosis. The High Chair, because of its back support, is especially helpful in rehabilitating weak or injured backs, as well as hip, knee or ankle injuries, and offers a good starter experience for those students who are new to exercise in general.

The Barrels

Joseph Pilates designed the Barrels – in their various forms – to develop and align the spine. The Barrels decompress the spine, promote its flexibility and develop the muscles surrounding it to be uniformly long, strong and stable. Pilates believed that everyone's spine has a natural, healthy alignment, but that everyday life works to destroy it. A healthy spine is central to a healthy mind and body; it enables you to move and breathe easily and powerfully, and it provides the central support for your body's limbs and organs. The exercises Joseph Pilates designed on the Barrels correct poor posture, open and stretch the chest, lengthen and strengthen the hips and hip flexors, massage the lower back and stretch and balance the legs.

Barrel work also develops strong abdominal muscles by requiring you to stabilize your Powerhouse. Barrel exercises stretch and strengthen the sides of the body to help you further strengthen your abdominal muscles and release tight lower-back muscles. Since the spine is rounded forwards, sideways or backwards over the curving surface of the Barrel during the exercises, Barrel work trains the abdominals in that unique Pilates way of developing length and strength simultaneously.

The Barrel comes in three basic designs: the High or Ladder Barrel, the Spine Corrector or Hump Barrel, and the Small Barrel.

The High or Ladder Barrel

The High/Ladder Barrel is the largest, approximately 1m (3ft) high and 23cm (21in) wide. A ladder, with four horizontal rungs and a wooden bottom brace attaches to one side of the barrel. The ladder rungs and brace provide hand- and foot-holds.

The main exercises on the High Barrel focus on leg stretching, sit-ups in all directions and spinal extension. The design of the equipment enables you to work on gentle backbends and simple exercises designed to eliminate hamstring tightness, or to work on more demanding exercises such as gymnastic walkovers and handstanding levitation.

The Spine Corrector

FIGURE 6-6

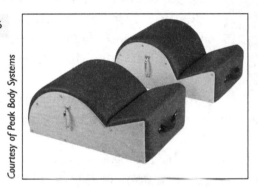

Courtesy of Peak Body Systems

The Spine Corrector (see FIGURE 6-6) is also known as the Hump Barrel, and does just what it's designed to do – correct imbalances or weaknesses in the spine. You do most of the exercises Pilates developed for this piece while lying with your back arched over the barrel. The Hump Barrel exercises stretch the tight muscles in the chest, shoulders, sides of the body and front of the hips – muscles that pull the spine out of correct alignment. The Hump Barrel helps you develop a more uniformly strong and supple spine by massaging, supporting and challenging your spine and Powerhouse muscles.

The Small Barrel

FIGURE 6-7

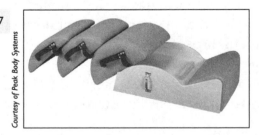

Courtesy of Peak Body Systems

Because Joseph Pilates understood there are so many different bodies with unique and special needs, he designed several versions of the Barrel. The Small Barrel, shown in FIGURE 6-7, is the simplest and most portable of his designs, yet with it you can achieve many of the valuable, essential Pilates movement goals – a flexible, decompressed spine; core power; and full-body uniform development. It's a great tool for your home studio. Imagine how good it would feel to lie back over it and stretch your arms, shoulders, chest and back after a long day at your computer or desk.

The Foot Corrector

FIGURE 6-8

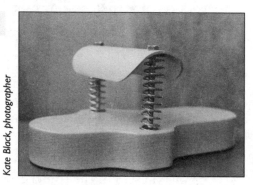

Kate Black, photographer

Unfortunately, we don't spend our days walking barefoot on sand or grassy earth that would massage and stretch our feet, toes, ankles and calves; instead, we stride quickly along hard, manufactured surfaces that pound, rather than develop, our joints and muscles.

Furthermore, few of us wear ideal footgear; our shoes constrict and weaken our feet, and prevent them from moving and developing in natural ways.

Joseph Pilates understood the value of having healthy, strong, flexible, balanced feet, and he designed one piece of equipment specifically for the purpose of developing them. The Foot Corrector is one of the smallest extant pieces of original Pilates equipment. It has a vaguely foot-shaped wooden base with a metal arch rising above it, supported by two heavy springs. (FIGURE 6-8 is a close-up of a Foot Corrector manufactured by Spenard Enterprises.)

To use the Foot Corrector, you stand over the apparatus and, with good Pilates body awareness and control, wrap one foot over the metal arch. You then use the muscles in your foot and lower leg to compress and release the spring. You can place your foot in several different positions on the metal arch, depending on the area of your foot that you'd like to strengthen, stretch and massage.

Don't dismiss the importance of healthy feet! When your feet and legs grow weak and tight, you feel tired all over. The Foot Corrector is designed to address this very basic and widespread problem. It can correct fallen arches, weak ankles, plantar fasciatis, bunions and more. The Foot Corrector also builds proper alignment of the foot, ankle, knee and hip joints – all of which help to provide you with better support as you stand, walk and sit.

The Ped-O-Pul

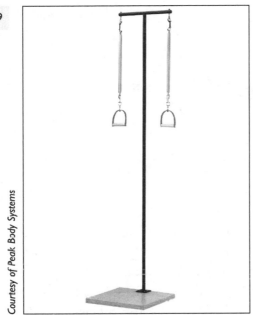

Courtesy of Peak Body Systems

Joseph Pilates designed the Ped-O-Pul specifically to help a famous opera singer learn how to breathe more effectively. This apparatus may not turn you into an opera star, but it can do a number of other equally wonderful things for you!

The Ped-O-Pul, shown in FIGURE 6-9, consists of a wooden base that measures about 46cm (18in) to 61cm (2ft) square, with a 2m (6.ft 6in) pole rising out of it along the back edge. A 46cm (18in) bar runs across the top of the pole, to form a T; and springs with handles hang from each end of the T-bar.

The entire Ped-O-Pul apparatus is freestanding and purposefully unstable. In most exercises, you stand with your back lightly touching the pole, and it becomes your job to stabilize it with your Powerhouse – a great tool for developing core strength and whole-body balance and awareness. All Ped-O-Pul exercises involve holding the spring handles and using the spring tension to elongate and stabilize your spine and Powerhouse; each exercise also demands that you balance the use of muscles across your shoulder girdle, to help strengthen and broaden your shoulders so you can stand and breathe more healthily.

The Ped-O-Pul is a valuable tool for repatterning poor neck and shoulder habits, and integrating your shoulder girdle movements to your core. Like all Pilates equipment, the Ped-O-Pul teaches full body coordination and control.

The Magic Circle

Joseph Pilates designed the Magic Circle (see Figure 6-10) to be versatile, lightweight and portable – perfect for use in the studio, at home and when travelling. Magic Circles come in several different strengths, depending on the number of layers of metal bands the Circle contains (the Magic Circle comes in two, three or four layers). These bands are held in place by two padded or upholstered grips.

FIGURE 6-10

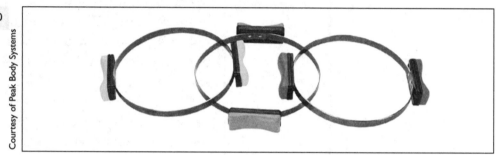

Courtesy of Peak Body Systems

You can use the Magic Circle to correct, reshape and strengthen various parts of your body, including the Powerhouse, inner thighs, arms, chest and neck. Regular work with the Magic Circle also helps to improve your posture and balance. You can position the hoop between your ankles, knees or hands, and then squeeze and release it with controlled motions. You can press the Magic Circle to your hip with your arm or hold it against your forehead or under your chin as you compress it. You press and release the Magic Circle while holding it above, in front of, or behind your body. You can use it while standing, sitting or lying down.

The Magic Circle is great in combination with other equipment, or when used to make mat-work exercises such as the Hundred, the Roll-U, or the Spine Stretch more challenging (you will learn about these exercises in later chapters).

The Beanbag

FIGURE 6-11

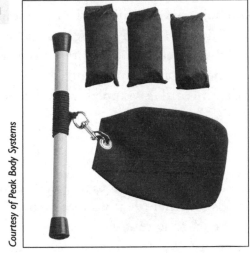

Courtesy of Peak Body Systems

The Beanbag (see FIGURE 6-11) is another piece of Pilates equipment that's small and portable, so you can use it at home, in the studio, at work or on the road. The Beanbag is an incredibly simple device, made up of a short length of thick, wooden dowel with the end of a long cord attached to its middle. At the other end of the cord hangs a bag of dried beans (1.5kg/3lb is a good weight). You use the Beanbag by holding the dowel with both hands and rolling it to raise and lower the weighted bag.

The Beanbag is designed to strengthen your arms and upper body, and to help tie this strength into that of your core muscles, thus providing a full-body workout. The Beanbag exercise offers an especially great way to rehabilitate shoulder, wrist and elbow injuries. If you suffer from carpal tunnel syndrome, tennis elbow or 'mouser's' shoulder, talk to your Pilates instructor or rehabilitation therapist about incorporating some Beanbag exercises into your rehabilitation programme.

Make Your Own Beanbag

As you've seen, the Beanbag design is simple and straightforward; in fact, you can easily make one of your own. You will need the following:

· 30–46cm (12–18in) section of a wooden dowel, 2.5cm (1in) in diameter or slightly larger
· 2m (6ft) clothesline or sturdy cord
· small cloth bag
· 1.5kg (3lb) dried beans

Drill a small hole through the middle of the dowel. Thread the cord through the hole and tie one end with a knot large enough to keep the cord from slipping through. If you don't have a drill, you can also staple or nail the cord to the middle of the dowel. The cord must be attached securely and unable to slip around the dowel as you turn it. Put the beans in the bag and tie the other end of the cord securely around the neck of the bag. Wind the dowel until the entire cord is wrapped around it. Now you have your own Beanbag.

The Beanbag Exercise

Stand with good Pilates posture – stomach scooped in and up the front of your spine; legs straight and heels together (gently squeeze together the entire inner line of both your legs throughout the exercise). Hold the Beanbag dowel straight out in front of you, hands on either side of the cord and the cord wrapped away from your body. Keep your shoulders down, elbows straight and unlocked, and wrists flat, as you gently stretch your knuckles away from your shoulder joints. Then follow these steps:

1. With precise control, slowly unwind the cord, lowering the beanbag towards the floor by simultaneously releasing your right hand and bending that wrist backwards as you curl your left hand forwards and away from you. As your right wrist bends backwards, the fingers of that hand reach for the ceiling; as your left hand curls forwards, those knuckles stretch towards the floor.

2. Grasp the dowel with your right hand, and repeat the curling and backward-bending motions, but with opposite hands (right hand curls forwards, left hand bends back). Remember to slowly stretch the fingers of your left hand down, then up, as the wrist bends backwards, as far as is comfortable for you. The knuckles of your right hand stretch away from your shoulders as they curl over and down towards the floor.

3. Breathe in and out with a natural rhythm, maintaining your scoop as you continue the alternating pattern, until the Beanbag reaches the floor (finish by holding the dowel in your left hand, which is

rotated down, knuckles pointing to the floor, with your right hand bent back at the wrist and fingers flared).

4. Now, begin another series of alternating curling and backward-bending motions, beginning by rotating the left wrist backwards, lifting the knuckles of your left hand to the ceiling. Simultaneously, reach forwards and down over the dowel with your right hand, knuckles curling towards the floor.

5. Grasp the dowel with the right hand and begin bending that hand backwards as your left hand releases and curls forwards, fingers stretching first towards the ceiling, then to the floor, as the hand reaches over to grasp the dowel.

6. Continue this alternating pattern until you've fully rewound the cord and the Beanbag reaches the dowel. Do this entire unwinding and winding sequence only once.

Be aware of your posture at all times during the Beanbag exercise (use a mirror if necessary). Stand with your feet rooted into the ground, keep your stomach scooped and your hips over your feet. Don't allow your pelvis to tuck or thrust forwards, and keep your shoulders down, your knees and elbows strong but unlocked. To get the most from this exercise, really work your forearms, wrists and hands, and articulate all the joints in your fingers as you unwind and wind the weighted bag. Imagine you're kneading dough or clay with the actions of your fingers and wrists.

If the exercise is too difficult for you initially, you have several options for modifying it; for example, you can reduce the weight of the bag, or eliminate the bag altogether, to concentrate on winding and unwinding the dowel with powerful, effective movements. Over time, you can slowly increase the weight of the bag to its full 1.5kg/3lb size. Alternatively, you can limit the length of cord you wind and unwind in the exercise, gradually extending the length over time. Eventually, when you can unwind and rewind the cord all the way to and from the floor, you'll need to stand on a step, a stool, or a chair to make use of all 2m (6ft) of cord. Ultimately, you can do this exercise three times.

The Wall

The Wall is an exercise rather than a piece of Pilates equipment, but it appears in this chapter because Joe Pilates cleverly designed this exercise to turn any stationary wall into a fitness apparatus. The Wall exercise can be done anywhere, with no special clothing and no special equipment – just locate a wall, and you're ready to go! Try it at work to help loosen a stiff and tired body, refresh a sluggish mind and lift sagging spirits.

To do the Wall, follow these steps:

1. Stand with your feet 25 to 30cm (10 to 12in) away from a wall, with your back touching the wall from your coccyx to the top of your shoulders and perhaps the back of your head. Keep your legs straight and squeezed together, knees unlocked, feet pressed firmly into the ground with heels touching and toes about 5cm (2in) apart. Let your arms hang loosely by your sides with the palms facing in.

2. Scoop your stomach in and up along the front of your spine to gently lengthen and press your back into and up along the wall (don't force this action by overtightening your buttock muscles). If your shoulders are too tight or your upper back too rounded to comfortably touch the back of your head to the wall, allow your head to float a centimetre or two away from the wall.

3. Inhale as you raise both arms forwards and as high above your head as you can while keeping your entire back touching the wall and your shoulders down (refer to FIGURE 6-12).

4. Exhale as you reach both arms wide and out to the side, palms facing forward, as they circle back down to your thighs. Repeat this arm circle movement two more times, then reverse the circles three times.

   With each repetition of the arm circles, note that your arms move more freely and with more range. Let the motions of your arms help facilitate full, deep Pilates breathing. Eventually, your arms may touch the wall above your head and slide along it as they circle.

5. After six arm circles, inhale and begin curling your head, neck and then spine (one vertebra at a time) off the wall; let your arms dangle and fall forwards as you round-curl your spine, allowing the weight of your

head to gently pull you over. Peel your back off the wall like a piece of tape, maintaining your scoop in order to help articulate each vertebra of your spine as you slowly release them, one by one, from the wall.

6. Exhaling, continue rounding forwards, stopping when you feel a comfortable amount of stretch in your back and/or hamstrings, keeping your lower pelvis stable against the wall. Finish exhaling as you reach the end of your forwards movement (your hands should be at least 20 to 25cm (8 to 10in) from the floor). Continue to maintain your scoop and keep your knees straight but unlocked. (See FIGURE 6-13.)

FIGURE 6-12

FIGURE 6-13

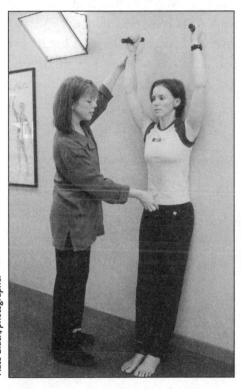
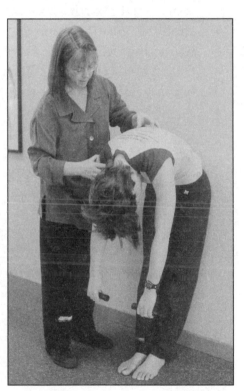

Kate Black, photographer

7. Continue breathing with a natural rhythm as you make small circles about the size of grapefruits with both arms. Each arm circles in the opposite direction from the other. Make eight to ten circles in one

direction, then reverse for eight to ten more, letting your arms slowly come to a stop.

8. Inhale smoothly and slowly, as you draw your stomach in and up the front of your spine to lengthen and place your spine, vertebra by vertebra, back up the wall, 'exactly in imitation of a wheel', as Joseph Pilates said.

9. Exhale as you continue to build your posture, stacking your vertebrae like building blocks, growing taller than you were when you began the exercise. Let your arms dangle and your shoulders settle easily on your torso as your upper back, neck and, possibly, head touch the wall in sequence.

When you finish the Wall, note how rejuvenated you feel. Your neck and shoulder tension is gone, your back feels long and relaxed, your hamstrings feel stretched and alive, and you're taller and breathing more fully! You can make the Wall work your muscles even more deeply by holding light weights or soup tins in your hands as you do the exercise.

CHAPTER 7

Introduction to
the Fundamental Skills
of Pilates

All Pilates exercises incorporate one or more of the seven fundamental movement skills described in this chapter. Together, these movement skills form a critical part of the entire Pilates system. In the next chapter, you will learn corresponding mini-exercises that will help you understand and develop these fundamental skills.

The Common Thread of Pilates Fundamental Skills

The fundamental skills of Pilates include understanding and controlling your range of motion in your pelvis, hip joint, ribcage or shoulder girdle/joint; awareness of effective body placement and position; the engagement of essential muscle groups for both movement and stabilization; and specific breathing techniques. By developing these fundamental skills, you form the basis upon which all Pilates exercises are built.

Promoting Uniform Development

Uniform development – a primary goal of Pilates – enables uniform nourishment. When your body is more uniformly developed, all its muscles, joints and organs receive ample amounts of healthy, oxygenated blood. Deep Pilates breathing helps bring that life-giving oxygen into your body, but in order for your circulation to carry oxygenated blood throughout your body, you must keep the paths open. You eliminate circulatory restrictions and constrictions by keeping all your muscles and joints equally strong and uniformly developed and your body well aligned.

Joseph Pilates knew that weak muscles and a stooped posture inhibit good circulation, and he developed his exercise system specifically to combat these physical shortcomings. Pilates also understood that a strong, well-aligned body does more with less effort. Strong muscles are flexible, responsive and promote good circulation, and they also keep the body upright, stable and well-balanced. Understanding the fundamental Pilates movement skills and their mini-exercises is your first step towards uniform development.

A Closer Look at the Body's Structure

Healthy muscle tone means that your musculature has appropriate firmness, consistency, elasticity and dimension, and, therefore, correctly conducts the electrical impulses from your nervous system that produce muscular activity and movement. Good tone in your muscles also promotes the circulatory system to do its job well and the skeletal structure to maintain its correct alignment.

FIGURE 7-1:
The skeletal
system

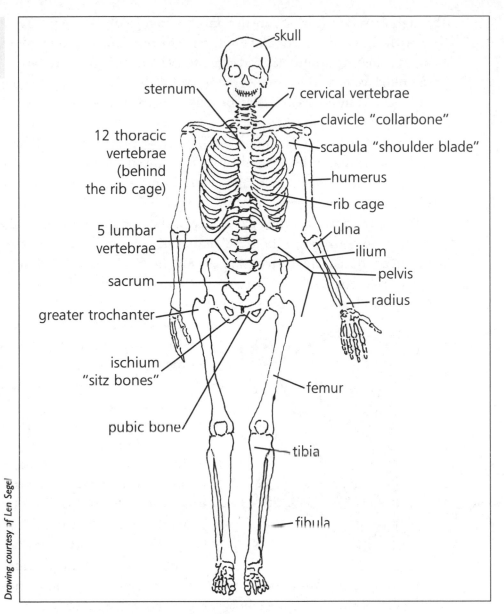

skull

sternum

7 cervical vertebrae

clavicle "collarbone"

scapula "shoulder blade"

12 thoracic
vertebrae
(behind
the rib cage)

humerus

rib cage

ulna

5 lumbar
vertebrae

ilium

pelvis

sacrum

radius

greater trochanter

ischium
"sitz bones"

femur

pubic bone

tibia

fibula

Imagine you're standing in a 'waterfall' of gravity and you're the funnel through which it reaches the earth. For a good, healthy, long life, your structure must be aligned and supported in such a way that you're completely in sync with this downward gravitational flow – at ease, and channelling the force effectively through your entire body, primarily through your bones, which are designed to do this job. When you're out of sync with the omnipresent and immutable force of gravity, you're slowly being crushed. Your muscles and other soft tissues are forced to bear misapplied weight, which makes them hard, tight and resistant to good circulation. Your bones, consequently, become weaker because they're not being required to hold you up.

However, when you're aligned with gravity, you can grow tall, using your bones and muscles to do the jobs they are supposed to do. Think about the redwood trees that can grow to hundreds of metres tall because they are in alignment with this powerful force.

To better appreciate the importance of the body's alignment, take a moment to consider the body's essential structure, as shown in the diagram of the skeletal system on page 87. (In this book you will see frequent references to specific bones and muscle groups; this diagram can help you locate the bones you read about.)

FIGURE 7-2:
The corset

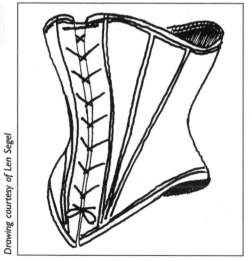

Drawing courtesy of Len Segel

You've seen the human skeleton depicted many times, but take a moment now to study the example offered here. Especially consider the large, open space between the base of the ribs and the pelvis – the section that houses many of your body's vital organs. No outside frame of bones provides structural support for the midsection of your body; that frame would inhibit your body's flexibility and mobility.

Instead, your spine provides the central support for your body's midsection, and your abdominal muscles are the corset that holds the whole thing together (see **FIGURE 7-2**).

The Abdominals

The abdominals are made up of four layers of powerful, elastic, crisscrossing bands of muscle fibres that give your body both stability and mobility. These muscles attach to your ribcage and your pelvis, and support your organs, spine and pelvis. This ever-important corset of abdominal support enables you to stand upright, to move your limbs and to expel air when you exhale. The abdominal muscles form the foundation of your body's powerful midsection – and are what many in Pilates refer to as your Powerhouse (see FIGURE 7-3). The four abdominal muscle groups are the *rectus abdominis,* the external obliques, the internal obliques and the *transversus abdominis.*

FIGURE 7-3:
Abdominal muscles

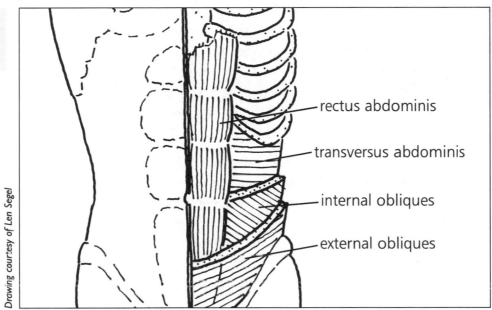

Drawing courtesy of Len Segel

rectus abdominis

transversus abdominis

internal obliques

external obliques

The *rectus abdominis* muscles run vertically up the front and centre of your body's midsection; they are the muscles that do crunches and (when well-developed) can give you that 'six-pack' so many people strive for. The *rectus abdominis* muscles primarily lift your upper body upright from a flat position, but are not effective in spinal stability, breathing or organ support. Pilates will teach you how to keep this muscle long when contracting it so it does not override the ability of the other abdominals to do their more important work.

The external and internal obliques are the two outer layers of the Powerhouse. Their diagonally crisscrossing fibres enable you to twist, flex and bend as they support your organs and stabilize your spine and pelvis.

To understand the importance of the conformation of your Powerhouse muscles, imagine how you would wrap an elastic bandage to support an injured knee. Stretching the bandage up and down along the front of the knee wouldn't provide adequate support. Crisscrossing the bandage around the knee gives the joint all-round, uniform support – the same way crisscrossed abdominals wrap and support your midsection.

The *transversus abdominis,* the deepest layer of abdominal muscles, consists of horizontal fibres that encircle the entire torso. This layer attaches to your diaphragm muscle and is primary to healthy breathing, organ support, and spinal and pelvic stability. Together, the *transversus* and obliques create the corset of power and support.

When the body is uniformly developed, the *transversus* fires first to stabilize the trunk before movement occurs. It is also the only abdominal muscle that is involved in moving the torso in every direction. Thus, the *transversus* is vital to your whole health, especially to long-lasting bones and joints.

In short, uniform development depends on powerful abdominal muscles that support a strong, stable spine. That's why the fundamental movement skills of Pilates focus on developing these physical attributes. The fundamental movement skills you learn here will help you master the Pilates method of body conditioning and add more years to your active, healthy life.

Pilates Breathing

Deep, healthy breathing is both a guiding principle and the first fundamental goal of Pilates. Joseph Pilates encouraged his students to 'above all, learn how to breathe correctly'. Deep breathing oxygenates your blood and sends it coursing throughout your system to nourish all your body's tissues. Pilates breathing contributes to a healthy body and an elevated mind and spirit.

What Happens When You Breathe?

If you're alive, you evidently know how to breathe, so why do you need to learn to breathe? You can train yourself to get more health benefit out of every breath you take, just as runners and power walkers improve upon the simple skills of running and walking learned as a child. In order to develop a better, healthier way of breathing, you first need to understand the basic physical process of breathing itself.

As you inhale, the intercostal muscles between your individual ribs contract to lift and widen your ribcage in a movement much like that of an umbrella beginning to open. At the same time, your diaphragm, the domelike muscle that attaches to the bottom of your lungs and separates your chest and abdominal cavities, contracts downwards, pulling your lungs with it. This action creates a vacuum that pulls air into your lungs. You then exhale by squeezing your *transversus abdominis,* which attaches all around the lower border of your ribcage, interweaving with the fibres of your diaphragm to pull the ribcage back down. This movement enables your diaphragm to relax and rise to its previous domed shape and expel the air from your lungs.

Effective, conscious breathing expands your lungs fully with each inhalation. Over time, ineffective or 'lazy' breathing overworks the more flexible parts of your lungs and allows the other areas to grow continually stiffer and tighter. Uniformly deep breathing leads to uniform development. First find the unexpanded areas of your lungs and teach them to stretch; that's how you can develop full-capacity breathing.

Pilates breathing is based on powerfully contracting and then expanding your lungs with each deep exhalation and inhalation. As Joseph Pilates advised, when you exhale, vigorously push all the air from your lungs, 'in much the same manner that you would wring every drop of water from a wet cloth'.

The Pilates Scoop

The Pilates scoop is the second fundamental movement skill of Pilates. The scoop is the powerful and eloquent action of drawing your abdominal wall in and up towards the front of your spine, thereby decompressing your spine and developing a strong Powerhouse or core. 'The Powerhouse' is a term used in Pilates to refer to the core of your body between your ribs and your hips and includes all four of your abdominal muscle groups. Three of these abdominal muscles completely surround your torso and attach through your lower back into your spine, creating a 'corset' or 'girdle' of strength and support. You use the fundamental movement skill of the Pilates scoop in every Pilates exercise to find your centre, to lengthen and stabilize your spine and torso and to balance your body, both in motion and at rest.

Pelvic Range of Motion

Even if you never do an advanced Pilates exercise, you can still benefit from knowing how to move your pelvis and lower spine correctly and healthily. The Pilates fundamental movement skill of pelvic range of motion trains your awareness and intentional use of the inherent, natural movement capabilities of your pelvis in relationship to your spine and legs.

Pilates gives you more choices in your movement patterns and habits, to halt repetitive-movement injuries and to build more uniform development that in turn, increases your stamina, your gracefulness and your whole body health. If you've ever hurt your lower back simply by bending over to pick something up, the value of this skill becomes apparent. Understanding pelvic movement will help you find correct ways of standing, lifting, sitting and moving, with less strain and wear and tear on your spine and lower-back muscles.

Each exercise in the Pilates method requires precise control of your pelvis and spine, and each is designed to balance your pelvis, so that it's properly oriented no matter what activity you're engaged in. If you have a natural tendency to tuck your pelvis, the exercises will stretch your hamstrings and lengthen your lower-abdominal muscles, and strengthen your lower back correctly, to increase the curve in your lumbar spine. If you arch your back too much, use the exercises to strengthen your abdominals and hamstrings in order to lengthen your lower back and pull your pelvis into the correct alignment. The movements and position of your pelvis and spine affect the stability and mobility of your entire body. Your ability to understand the fundamental movement skill of pelvic range of motion will help you achieve uniform development – and a longer, healthier life.

The Pelvic Rocking mini-exercise you will learn in the next chapter will teach you how your pelvis and lumbar spine move through flexion and extension, how far is a healthy end range, and what the ripple effect of pelvic movement is on the rest of the body. Moving too far, not far enough, or using the wrong muscles to create the movement can lead to inefficiency or – even worse – strain and injury.

Pelvic Stability

Now that you've familiarized yourself with the fundamental movement skills of Pilates breathing, Pilates scoop and pelvic range of motion, you're ready to coordinate them into a new, more complicated skill that is equally fundamental to all Pilates exercises – pelvic stability.

In everyday activities, if your pelvis and spine rock and shift inappropriately as you raise and lower your legs, you can strain or even injure the muscles in your hips and lower back. By keeping your pelvis appropriately stable and still during movements involving hip flexions and extensions, you avoid the risks of muscle strain and injury.

The pelvic stability movement may be carried out through a mini-exercise called Knee Folds (see Chapter 8), in which you stabilize your pelvis and spine against the movement and weight of your legs. This strengthens your abdominals and teaches you how to keep your *rectus abdominis* muscle long, even as you engage it, so it doesn't crunch and limit the effectiveness of the other three abdominal groups as they work to stabilize your spine and pelvis.

Building Pelvic Stability

Pelvic stability is the fundamental skill of stabilizing your pelvis against the movement of your legs and spine so that you don't pull on your spine or hips as you walk, run, climb stairs, bend, twist, push and lift. Your scooped abdominals stabilize your pelvis and spine, giving you better access to your deep hip flexor muscles – the *iliopsoas* – so you can move your leg safely and efficiently. If your body or your movements are out of balance, external flexors such as the *rectus femoris* (located on the front of your thigh) override the *iliopsoas*, leading to overworked quads and underdeveloped deep hip flexors. This can put strain on your body and lead to inefficiency or injury.

The *iliopsoas* is really made up of two sets of muscles – the *psoas* and the *iliacus*. The *psoas* attaches at each vertebra along the front and sides of your lumbar spine and joins with the *iliacus* that lines the inside of your pelvic bones. Together, these muscles pass through your pelvis and insert onto the inside of the top of your femur.

The *iliopsoas* has two very important jobs: to pull your thigh bone to your spine when your spine is stabilized, and to pull your spine to your thigh when your legs are stabilized.

You call upon this muscle group often in Pilates – and in life. Because these muscles attach to your spine, pelvis and legs, learning to move these parts of your body correctly, both independently and in relationship to one another, requires some practice – but it's a skill well worth learning. You must be able to maintain a stable pelvis and spine as you flex your hip, to avoid straining your back or damaging your hip, a skill you will learn by practising Knee Folds.

Spinal Twisting

Spinal twisting challenges you to stabilize your upper spine and shoulders as you twist your lower spine, pelvis and legs as one unit.

Spinal twisting stretches and strengthens your Powerhouse, and massages your back and abdominal muscles, ligaments, organs and even your spinal cord, stimulating your mind/body connection. Being able to distinguish between pelvic stability and spinal twisting will give you better control over your movements, and will enable your mind to be more precise in its directions. In this way, you move with more efficiency, which leads to better endurance and less chronic wear and tear or injury.

Although pelvic stability and spinal twisting deal with stabilizing one part of your body as other parts move, each requires a different set of muscular skills and movement control. Pay close attention to the different skills you use when performing Knee Sways (see Chapter 8), as opposed to Knee Folds.

Ribcage Stability

Ribcage stability is another skill that is fundamental to all Pilates exercises and movements. The mini-exercise Ribcage Arms, described in Chapter 8, involves stabilizing your spine and ribcage as you move your arms and shoulder girdle in a broad, controlled motion. Mastering the skill of ribcage stabilization will give your arms and shoulders their widest range of safe, healthy motion, enabling you to reach and lift away from your body without suffering muscle strain or injury.

Understanding Your Shoulder's Anatomy

The shoulder is a complex mechanical structure made up of two distinct yet interrelated skeletal parts: the shoulder girdle and the arm. The shoulder girdle includes the collarbone (clavicle) and the shoulder blade (scapula); the upper arm bone (humerus) attaches to the shoulder blade to form the shoulder joint. The entire arm and shoulder girdle unit connects to the rest of the skeleton at the breastbone (sternum) and rests on top of the ribcage.

The unique design of this mechanism provides your arm and shoulder with a tremendous range of motion. But this capability also sets the stage for a number of potentially damaging movement habits and the injuries that result from this extended range of motion. Many people develop severely limiting shoulder injuries by overextending the humerus in its joint – sometimes even dislocating it. Injuries such as torn rotator cuffs commonly result from allowing the muscles surrounding the joint to become imbalanced.

Just because a movement is natural doesn't necessarily mean that your body will automatically 'know' and follow that movement. Physical imbalances and long-term movement habits can make inefficient – even damaging – movements seem quite normal. The movements and exercises you learn in this book help you retrain your body to its true (and healthy) natural movement style.

Injuries also result from failing to articulate the motion of the shoulder, by moving the shoulder girdle and humerus as one, rather than as individual parts. This problem can lead to imbalanced use of the neck and shoulder muscles and improper timing of the movement of the humerus in its joint. This lack of uniform development can result in overuse injuries such as bursitis and tendonitis, 'tennis elbow' or carpal tunnel and thoracic outlet syndromes. Balancing the muscle movements surrounding your arm and shoulder girdle is essential to maintaining a strong, healthy, pain-free shoulder.

There is an inherent, natural rhythm involved in the engagement of muscles as they move the arm and shoulder girdle. We often destroy this natural rhythm with poor movement habits. Retrieving those lost, naturally efficient muscle-firing patterns begins with learning to stabilize your ribcage and spine. Learning proper shoulder range of motion and ribcage stabilization teaches you healthy movement and corrects damaging movement habits.

Upper Spinal Flexion

Upper spinal flexion is the most challenging of all the fundamental movement skills discussed in this chapter and requires the most abdominal strength. Performing the Upper Body Curl mini-exercise (described in the next chapter) teaches this skill as it builds the strong abdominal muscles and a healthy range of motion in your upper spine. You must be capable of using your Powerhouse to support and lift the entire weight of your head, shoulders, and upper body from a supine position (lying on your back) in a controlled, precise and flowing movement. In addition, you must stabilize your pelvis and lower spine, restricting the tendency of those strong muscles to work inappropriately.

When you perform the upper spinal flexion, you need to rely on all the other fundamental movement skills that you've learned in this chapter. Pilates breathing stretches your ribcage and middle and upper back as it strengthens your Powerhouse. The Pilates scoop trains your abdominal corset to stay long and strong while it works. The pelvic range of motion teaches you awareness and control of your pelvic range of motion. The pelvic stability you will develop through practising Knee Folds will make the upper spinal flexion a safer, more powerful movement. And you'll definitely call upon the 'body knowledge', balance, flexibility and control you will have gained by moving and stabilizing your spine, arms and pelvis through the spinal twisting and ribcage stability mini-exercises.

Finding Your Fundamental Mat Posture

To get the most from any Pilates exercise, you first must focus your mind, explore and discover your own body's capabilities and inherent strengths and weaknesses, and find an effective pelvic and spinal alignment. Follow these simple steps to begin your exploration and to find an effective fundamental mat posture:

1. Start by lying down on the mat, flat on your back, knees bent, feet flat and legs hip-width apart, arms resting along your sides with

palms turned down. Your heels will be about 25 to 30cm (10 to 12in) away from your sitz bones.

2. Begin training your awareness and concentration principles; relax all your muscles and scan your whole body for any tension or resistance. Notice what part of your back (spine, ribs and pelvis) touches the mat and decide where you feel your weight resting on the mat. If you have a mirror, look to see how your body lies on the mat.

3. Gently rock your pelvis forwards and backwards 10 or 12 times to help release any tightness, and note how your weight shifts. Allow your whole spine and even your head to be rocked by this movement. Then find the lower back and spinal position that feels the most comfortable with the least amount of muscle resistance or activity. This is your fundamental mat posture.

Note where your weight rests now. Is it different from the way it rested when you first lay down on the mat? Has your spine become more elongated, your lower back or neck closer or further from the floor, your back more relaxed, your ribcage softened or settled? Each time you begin your mat-work session, follow these steps to arrive at this posture anew. The mat should be supporting your spine, head, legs, arms, hands and feet comfortably. If necessary, try some of these tips for easing into the position:

·   If you feel any shoulder or neck strain, or if your head feels as if it has to reach too far back to be able to rest on the mat, place a small pillow under your head.

·   If your feet slip on the mat, remove your socks or position yourself so that your feet are propped or supported by a wall or piece of furniture.

·   If you can't straighten your arms comfortably with your palms down, try turning them face up.

The neutral pelvis position you arrive at today is a good starting position for the mini-exercises that follow in the next chapter. Expect this posture to evolve with you every day, as your regular Pilates practice develops your body's strength, length, balance and flexibility.

CHAPTER 8

Fundamental Skills Mini-Exercises

In Chapter 7, you went over the seven fundamental movement skills of Pilates. In this chapter, mini-exercises allow you to practise these movement skills. If you're weak or recovering from injury, practising these mini-exercises will help you build uniform strength, flexibility and stability, and will develop your awareness and control of your body.

Practise Your Pilates Breathing

This mini-exercise teaches proper Pilates breathing. It follows the natural breathing process the human body experiences every day, but it teaches you more conscious control, it expands your lung capacity, and it strengthens all the muscles you use to breathe. This, in turn, cleanses and detoxifies your body.

1. Lie in your fundamental mat posture and begin by inhaling through your nose (mouth closed, but relaxed), expanding your lungs as far as you can in all directions. As you inhale, feel your ribs inflate and expand, and your stomach scoop in and up. As you breathe in, feel your ribs expanding and widening in every direction, your diaphragm contracting and lowering, and your lungs pulling air in. (See FIGURE 8-1.)

2. Exhale with an open mouth and slowly and steadily draw in your abdominal muscles to squeeze the air from your lungs. Make the squeezing movements completely encircle your torso, so your front, sides and lower back work in unison. Don't tense or grip your muscles to exhale; instead, contract your abdominal muscles strongly, elastically and evenly expelling all of the air in your lungs out through your open

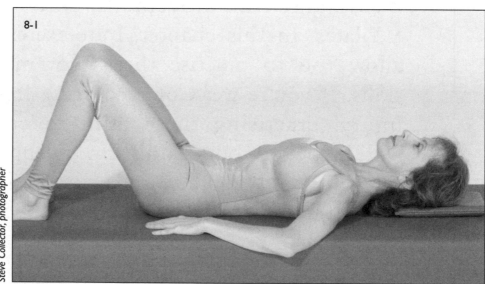

8-1

Steve Collector, photographer

mouth. When you exhale fully, your waist narrows and the distance between your ribs and hips lengthens all the way around your body.

3. Repeat this deep Pilates breathing mini-exercise four or five times, each time attempting to pull more air into your lungs and squeeze more air out of them.

Use the guiding principle of concentration and awareness to develop your Pilates breathing technique. As you inhale and exhale fully, use your mind's eye to follow the breath into and out of your lungs, and be aware of where your breath easily goes – and where it seems to stop.

Tips for Developing Your Pilates Breathing

As you work on your Pilates breathing skill, remember the goal of uniform development. You want your lungs to fully expand in all directions simultaneously and readily, as they are designed to do. Explore the feeling of expanding your lungs into different places in your chest and upper back. Try 'breathing' into your armpits, under your collarbone or sternum, between your shoulder blades, into your mid-back or down into your stomach. When you find a part of your body that doesn't seem to expand to accommodate your lungs, practise inflating that area several times in a row. Using your awareness when practising your breathing enables you to discover areas that lack uniform development and to learn to fully expand your ribcage and lungs with your breath consistently from one area to the next. Access to the entire capacity of your lungs is essential to your health.

Note that when you expand your stomach as you breathe, your lungs don't expand as fully everywhere else. To uniformly develop your breathing capacity (and strengthen your core muscles), scoop your abdominals in and up to limit the amount of breath that expands your stomach. This approach encourages your lungs to expand more fully into your ribcage and back, stretching you from the inside out, and it gives you more immediate access to your full lung capacity.

Before moving on to the next fundamental skill, check for any changes in your fundamental mat posture. Have more parts of your back released or settled into the mat? Has your weight distribution changed?

Practise Your Pilates Scoop

To perform the Pilates scoop, lie down on your back, assuming your fundamental mat posture. Then, follow these steps:

1. As you exhale, draw your abdominal muscles away from your pubic bone, in towards your spine and up under your ribs, creating a deep, hollow, scooped-out bowl in your abdomen. This is a muscular action only – don't move your pelvis or spine. This action strengthens your abdominal muscles while maintaining their length, but only if you keep your pelvis and spine still.
2. Inhale, maintaining the scoop.
3. Exhale even more powerfully to deepen this squeezing, scooping action.
4. Do this mini-exercise three or four more times to get your Powerhouse muscles firing powerfully. Be sure to keep your neck and shoulders relaxed.

Practise Your Pilates Scoop with Pilates Breathing

When you become comfortable with the Pilates skill of scooping, add the full breath cycle of the Pilates breathing mini-exercise. As you practise the following mini-exercise of scooping with Pilates breathing, notice how the scoop limits the expansion of your abdomen and thereby encourages your breath to more fully enter and expand your lungs.

1. Lie in your fundamental mat posture. Exhale fully, then slowly inhale through your nose, inflating your lungs and ribcage in every direction. Allow that widening, lengthening feeling to help draw your abdominals deeply in and up along the front of your spine, like the undertow of a wave. As your ribcage expands, your waist gets narrower, like the middle of an hourglass.

2. Open your mouth and exhale completely, drawing the strings of your corset as tightly as possible. Expel all your air to create a vacuum in your lungs.

3. Repeat steps 1 and 2 three or four more times, deepening your scoop and increasing your breathing capacity and your exhaling power with each repetition.

Tips for Developing Your Scoop

When you perform the scoop, think about the encircling corset of muscles surrounding your Powerhouse, and draw the corset strings tight around your waist. Feel how the scoop creates powerful support for your organs and spine, and thereby forms a strong foundation to support the movement of your limbs.

Pelvic Rocking Mini-Exercise

Follow these steps of the Pelvis Rocking mini-exercise (SEE FIGURE 8-2) to learn how your pelvis moves from a curl through a neutral posture into an arch, and what is a safe range of motion for you today:

1. Lie in your fundamental mat posture and press your feet down into the mat and slightly back towards your hips (without moving them).

2. To begin curling your pelvis off the mat, draw your hamstring muscles up the back of your thighs towards your knees as you scoop your abdominals in and up the front of your spine. As your

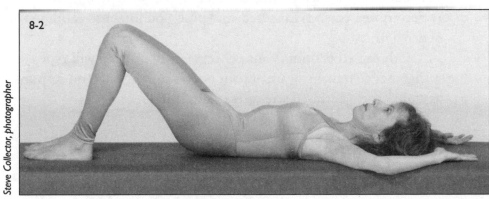

8-2

Steve Collector, photographer

hamstrings contract, allow them to gently pull your sitz bones with them off the mat, curling your pelvis away from your body. This is a very small movement; only until your sitz bones are about 5 or 7.5cm (2 or 3in) off the mat, the healthy end-range of pelvic motion in the curl phase of the Pelvic Rocking mini-exercise. In the curl phase, your lower back is decompressed and your abdominals are scooped.

To get the most from this phase of the Pelvic Rocking mini-exercise, keep these points in mind:

- As your sitz bones rise away from you, your lower back lengthens and moves closer to (or perhaps even touches) the mat. Your pelvis, sacrum and lumbar vertebrae sequentially elongate and articulate, curling off the mat until you reach your waist. Don't pull your pubic bone back towards you or press your lower back into the mat.
- Allow the lengthening of your pelvis away from your ribcage to scoop your abdominals up along the front of your spine.
- Keep your knees 7.5 or 10cm (3 or 4in) apart; keeping good leg alignment during the curl engages your hamstrings and inner thighs.

In a curl, your body is gently elongated on a shallow diagonal towards your knees – stretched like soft toffee. This movement should feel great. Your lower back should be gently flexed, lengthened and relaxed; your abdominals stretched and gently scooped; and your spine decompressed. If you crunch your abdominals, contract your back or grip your gluteals, you will inappropriately shorten (tuck) rather than lengthen (curl). A curl is decompressed and elongated, and pulls you into a streamlined, centred unity.

With each repetition, your pelvic range of motion will evolve, so remember to remain aware of your body's capabilities and responses as it develops increased strength and balance.

The Arch

The second step of the Pelvic Rocking mini-exercise is to move into the arch:

1. Sequentially roll your lumbar spine, sacrum and pelvis down onto the mat, lengthening your hamstrings and lowering your sitz bones.
2. Maintain your abdominal scoop as you continue to rotate your pelvis away from you until your pubic bone, coccyx and sitz bones are pointing on a long shallow diagonal towards your heels. Your lower back is gently extended and arched away from the mat. As with the curl, this is a very small movement. This is your healthy end-range of pelvic motion in the arch phase of the Pelvic Rocking mini-exercise (see FIGURE 8-3).

In the arch phase of the Pelvic Rocking mini-exercise, remember the following points:

·   Don't strain, crunch, push or overextend your lower back up off the mat in your arch. Even in extension (arch), your spine is long and decompressed.
·   Maintain your scoop even as your pelvis rotates away.
·   Allow the movement to gently shift your ribs, neck and head, but in a very small range.

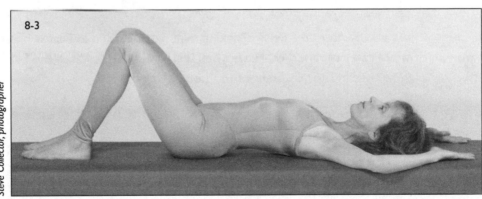

8-3

Steve Collector, photographer

The Neutral Posture

Finally, to find your neutral posture, continue with these steps:

1. Rock gently back and forth between the arch and the curl five or six times.
2. Continue your Pilates breathing and scoop, and make the rocking movement smaller and smaller, until you find a still pelvic posture somewhere equally balanced between the arch and curl. This is your healthy neutral pelvic posture today. In neutral, your pubic bone and hipbones are approximately level with each other and parallel to the mat.

Tips for Developing Pelvic Range of Motion

As you move through the curl, arch and neutral phases of the Pelvic Rocking mini-exercise, be aware of which phase feels the most comfortable and familiar to your body. You can also find some important clues to your body's natural pelvic placement by standing in front of a mirror and assessing your posture. Do you overarch your back, consequently promoting weak abdominal muscles and a tight lower back? Or do you tend to stand with your pelvis tucked under? That posture leads to short, tight hamstrings and an overstretched, unstable lumbar region. Either of these postures indicates that your body isn't uniformly developed.

As you perform the Pelvic Rocking mini-exercise, add in Pilates breathing and Pilates scoop to challenge your skills and build towards the Pilates exercises in later chapters of this book.

Performing the Knee Folds

This exercise improves your pelvic stability. To correctly stabilize your pelvis, you engage your abdominal corset and the muscles surrounding your pelvis, including your gluteals, inner thighs, pelvic floor, deep hip rotators and hamstrings, just enough to do the job that is required – not too much and not too little. In the case of Knee Folds, you will need one level of stabilization when you lift one leg at a time, and greater stabilization when you lift both legs off the mat. This pelvic stabilization action is purely muscular and does not move your bones. In other words, you maintain a neutral pelvic posture. Don't arch or curl your pelvis as you lift or lower your legs.

To do the Knee Folds mini-exercise, follow these steps:

1. Lie in your fundamental mat posture, and this time gently squeeze your legs and feet together. Engage the muscles of your corset and pelvis to stabilize as you prepare to move.

2. Inhale with deep Pilates breathing, allowing the air to expand your ribs in all directions, lengthening your scoop up under the ribcage like the undertow of a wave. Use this lengthening of your scoop to lift one leg and crease it deeply at the hip joint as you fold your knee in towards your chest (see FIGURE 8-4). Imagine you're balancing a full teacup on your pubic bone to keep your pelvis still, and be careful not to spill the tea as you move your leg.

   Use precise control as you perform Knee Folds. Maintain a neutral pelvis (no curling or arching) and your scoop, lengthening your abdominals so they help stabilize your pelvis and spine against the weight of your moving leg. Don't allow your *rectus abdominis* muscles to shorten (making your belly bulge).

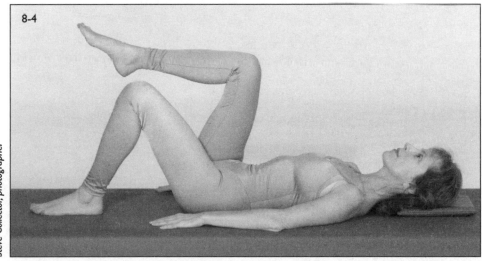

8-4

Steve Collector, photographer

Continue with the following steps:

3. Exhale, clinching your corset to maintain a stable pelvis as you lower your leg to the mat.
4. Repeat steps 1 to 3 four times with the same leg. Switch to your other leg, and repeat the movement five times.

Expanding Your Skills with Knee Folds

The more controlled and precise your Knee Folds are, the better grasp you have on pelvic stability, and the better you'll perform all the exercises you learn in this book. Mastering pelvic stability benefits more than your Pilates practice; it helps in all the movements of your life, including running, walking, lifting, bending, climbing stairs and more.

When you've become comfortable with the Knee Fold mini-exercise, experiment with reversing the breath pattern; exhale as you fold your bent leg into your chest, and inhale as you lower it back to the mat. With this breathing pattern, you can use the movement of folding your leg into your torso to assist in squeezing the air from your lungs as you exhale. Keep your scoop, especially as you inhale to lower your leg. And keep your pelvis stable. Do this version of Knee Folds four times, then repeat with the other leg.

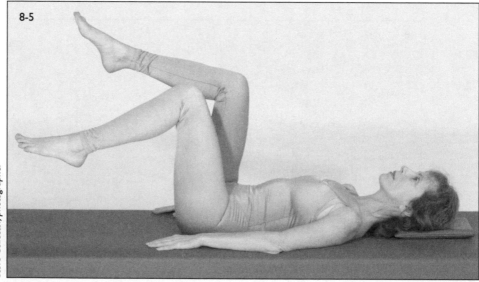

8-5

Steve Collector, photographer

Here's another variation on Knee Folds that further challenges your body and mind:

1. After you've folded your right leg to your chest as you inhaled, stay in this position as you exhale, stabilizing your pelvis even more deeply with your abdominal corset and pelvic muscles. Use oppositional energy to reach your sitz bones away from your ribcage so you don't tuck.

2. Inhale, deepening your scoop as you lift your left leg up to meet the right (see FIGURE 8-5). As you perform this variation, make sure you don't allow your pelvis to curl up off the mat, your abdominals to shorten or your back to arch, any of which will cause you to lose the support of your Powerhouse. Note that this version of the Knee Folds mini-exercise forces you to work harder to keep your pelvis stable and your abdominal muscles long and scooped.

3. Exhale to draw your corset strings snug, and engage the muscles around the base of your pelvis to further stabilize your pelvis. (When you stabilize your pelvis and spine correctly and powerfully as you lift your leg, you train the *iliopsoas* muscle to perform its vital task of flexing the hip efficiently and effectively.)

4. Inhale, scooping in your stomach even deeper, as you lower your right foot as low as you can without moving your spine or pelvis. Keep your knee bent.

5. Exhale, drawing the corset strings tighter, to fold your leg – creased at the hip – back to your chest. Don't tuck.

6. Repeat steps 4 and 5 with the left leg. Do three sets of this alternating leg pattern.

Every time you do this version of Knee Folds, start with a different leg, to promote uniform development. If you can't maintain pelvic stability or if your lower back tires when you do the more advanced version of the Knee Folds mini-exercise, lessen the range of motion and/or stop. When you do this version of Knee Folds correctly, your abdominals should tire before your back.

Working on Your Knee Sways

Knee Sways are one of the most effective mini-exercises for developing the fundamental Pilates skill of spinal twisting. Because your abdominals are attached to both your ribs and your pelvis, they are simultaneously strengthened and stretched by the movement of your knees in opposition to the stability of your shoulders and ribs. This spinal twisting skill is fundamental to many Pilates exercises as well as the movements you perform in daily activities.

Follow these steps to perform Knee Sways:

1. Lie in your fundamental mat posture, gently squeezing your legs and feet together; your knees and ankle bones are touching and should remain so throughout this exercise.

2. Inhale and scoop your stomach in and up your spine as you slowly sway both knees to the right, keeping your ribs and shoulders anchored to the mat and your knees and ankle bones gently pressed together. As your knees sway to the right, allow the weight of your knees to pull your pelvis into a slight twist, lifting the left hip off the mat. This movement should be small, controlled and flowing, with your abdominals constantly scooping in opposition to the weight of your lower body. Your left foot will rise off the mat, but your legs shouldn't shift or slide against each other. (See FIGURE 8-6.)

3. Exhale and scoop as you return your spine – vertebra by vertebra – lightly back to the mat, continuing until your spine, pelvis and legs return you to your neutral fundamental mat posture. (See FIGURE 8-7.)

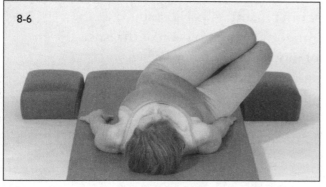

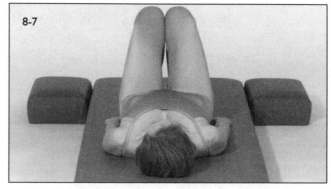

Steve Collector, photographer

Repeat steps 1 to 3, to the left. Alternate this twisting movement for three more sets of right and left; with each repetition and each set, try to increase your ability to twist your spine, move from your centre and strengthen your Powerhouse. Take a moment to notice and enjoy your newly found spinal range of motion. With each repetition, your spine will become springier.

Getting the Most from Knee Sways

Feel each vertebra as it rolls off and on the mat during Knee Sways, and allow your spine and pelvis to pass through a gentle pelvic curl in both directions as you twist and untwist. Don't press your back into the mat or grip your gluteals.

Use the concept of oppositional energy to stretch your squeezing inner thighs away from your scooping stomach during Knee Sways; this action decompresses your spine and pelvis and deepens your scoop.

When you do Knee Sways effectively, you feel a stretch in your waist, hips, outer thighs, lower back or deep stomach. Enjoy that stretch – it's a sign that your skills at spinal twisting are improving with each repetition.

Ribcage Arms Mini-Exercise

The Ribcage Arms mini-exercise involves training your abdominals to stabilize your ribcage and spine as you move your arm and shoulder girdle, and is designed to reveal and correct unhealthy movement habits.

To perform the Ribcage Arms mini-exercise, follow these steps:

1. Lie in your fundamental mat posture, feet flat on the floor and legs and feet gently squeezing together.
2. Inhale and scoop as you raise your arms towards the ceiling, perpendicular to the floor, palms facing each other (see FIGURE 8-8). Use your abdominal corset to effectively stabilize your ribcage. Keep your shoulder blades on the mat.
3. Exhale as you slowly lower your arms towards the mat above your head until you feel your shoulder blades beginning to slide down your back; at this point you've reached the end of your shoulder joint's

range of motion (the actual true range of your humerus in its socket), but your shoulder girdle can still move a bit farther.

4. Continue moving both your arms back and your shoulder blades down until any further movement would cause your ribs or chest to lift. This is as far as you can move your shoulder girdle safely (see FIGURE 8-9). Use your scooped abdominals and the power of your exhalation to keep your ribs from rising or lifting off the mat – in other words, to maintain ribcage stability. If you move your arms too far back your ribs will lift and your spine will arch, as shown in FIGURE 8-10. Make sure to keep elbows and wrists straight, but not locked, throughout the mini-exercise to get the stretch necessary to increase your range of movement over time.

5. Inhale, using your scooped abdominals to stabilize your spine and ribcage as you bring your arms back up to the ceiling.

6. Repeat steps 3 to 5 three more times. Each time, increase your ability to maintain ribcage and spinal stabilization to enable you to develop a larger safe range of motion in your arm and shoulder girdle over a period of time.

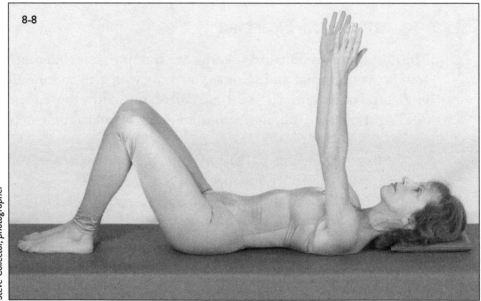

8-8

Steve Collector, photographer

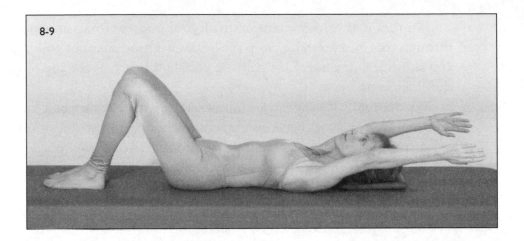

8-9

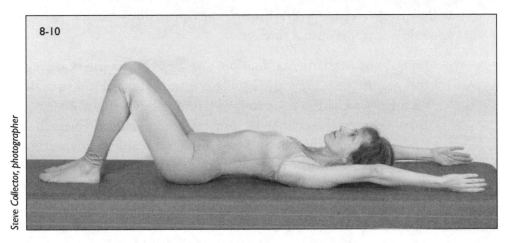

8-10

Steve Collector, photographer

If at any time you feel any tightness or restriction in your movements during the Ribcage Arms mini-exercise, exhale an extra time or two at that moment. Exhaling helps to release any unconscious tensing or holding back that might be preventing the safe, flowing movement of your arm and shoulder.

Tips for Getting the Most from Ribcage Arms

Use the Pilates guiding principle of concentration and awareness to note changes in your shoulder's true safe range of motion with each Ribcage Arms repetition.

For that matter, pay attention to all your body's signals as you work through this mini-exercise. Stop the backward movement of your arms and shoulders if you feel any pain – especially a pinch at the top of your shoulder joint.

Try doing the Ribcage Arms mini-exercise with one arm at a time, and note any discrepancies between the movement and range of motion in one arm and shoulder versus the other. Awareness of these imbalances will promote uniform development over time.

Performing the Upper Body Curl

Follow these steps to work through the Upper Body Curl, which develops your skill at upper spinal flexion:

1. Lie in your fundamental mat posture, feet flat on the floor, legs and feet gently squeezed together. Place your hands behind your head, resting its weight in your cupped palms, elbows slightly forwards.
2. Inhale deeply, then clinch in your corset to exhale as you pull your ribs, spine and upper body away from your stable pelvis, curling your head, shoulders, then upper body off the mat like a cresting wave (see FIGURE 8-11). In fact, imagine that your torso and upper body are a swelling, curling ocean wave rising over a surfer. The bottom tips of your shoulder blades remain touching the mat. As your wave crests over the surfer in the Upper Body Curl mini-exercise, use oppositional energy to draw your pelvis away from your ribs (see FIGURE 8-12).

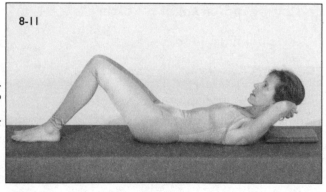
8-11

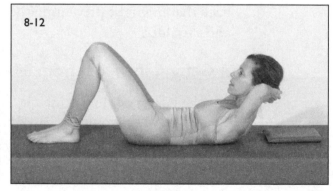
8-12

Steve Collector, photographer

3. Exhale as you suspend your curl, then inhale, experimenting with where to 'put' your breath. For example, inflate your lungs into your upper spine and the back of your ribs, to stretch your upper back even further away from your scooped abdominals. This action pulls your stomach and spine like soft toffee away from your hips.

4. Exhale, further lengthening your spine as you squeeze and elongate your Powerhouse. Allow that lengthening action to lower your upper body – one vertebra at a time – back down to and along the mat.

5. Repeat steps 2 to 4 three or four more times. With each repetition, lengthen your torso and spine further away from your pelvis, so that each time you roll your upper body back down you're taller than you were the previous time.

In the Upper Body Curl, stabilize your neutral pelvis further by scooping your abdominals deeply in and up the front of your spine and engaging your pelvic floor muscles, inner thighs, deep hip rotators, lower gluteals and upper hamstring muscles. Imagine that you're pulling these muscles away from your curl as you raise your upper body from the mat. Don't tuck or arch.

Gaining Skill with the Upper Body Curl

The Upper Body Curl is a difficult and complex mini-exercise. You can modify it with one of the following changes:

1. Lift your upper body less far off the mat.
2. Place one hand behind your head to help hold the weight of your head, reaching the other arm down along your side a couple of centimetres off the floor.

The second modification cuts down on the effort required of your abdominal muscles, so you can elongate your *rectus abdominis* more and scoop your stomach deeper. Deepening your scoop builds the strength and control you'll need to eventually be able to curl without assistance.

A correct Upper Body Curl is powerful; during it, your body's joints and muscles are decompressed, long and well-articulated. Here are some images that can help you attain this standard:

- Imagine that your torso and upper body are a swelling, curling ocean wave. Inherent in this image is the power of the wave's undertow – the deep abdominal scooping action that pulls your stomach in and up along the front of your spine and continues up into the curl.
- Imagine that your spine and upper body are coiling like a nautilus shell or a cinnamon roll.
- Imagine that the curling motion of your upper body is similar to that of a poster you're rolling to fit into a tube. You first sweep the poster's leading edge back and under, and then curl it forward over itself as you roll it. That's the way your spine moves in the Upper Body Curl.
- As you perform the Upper Body Curl, remember the Pilates guiding principles of concentration and awareness, precise control and flowing natural movements. Keep your upper back, neck and head aligned to make a uniform curve throughout your upper body. Move your head in concert with your spine, and then lift your entire upper body with your abdominals. Don't try to pull your head up by reaching forward with your face, nose or shoulders; you'll overstretch and strain your neck at the expense of building true core strength. (See FIGURE 8-13.) Remember: you're curling your spine, not heaving your head off the mat.

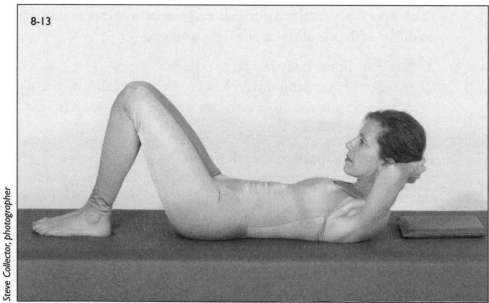

8-13

Steve Collector, photographer

Before Going on to Mat-Work Exercises

As you've learned in each of the preceding sections, your body will grow stronger, more balanced and capable as you gain practice in Pilates. So remember that your mastering of the fundamental skills of Pilates movement learned in this chapter will remain a work in progress.

Be true to your present fitness level and capabilities. Don't criticize or condemn. Know that your technique with each of these movements will change and grow over time; that kind of evolution is central to the practice and philosophy of the Pilates method of body conditioning. By being honest with yourself and allowing the process to unfold, you guarantee that Pilates will continue to offer you a safe, lifelong method for remaining healthy, fit and vital.

'Conscientiously, faithfully and without deviation... keep your mind wholly concentrated on the purpose of the exercises as you perform them.'

Joseph Pilates, *Your Health*

CHAPTER 9
The Pilates Hundred

The Hundred, one of the most fundamentally important of the Pilates method exercises, kicks off the series of mat-work exercises you will follow in Chapters 9–19. It was the first exercise Joseph Pilates described in *Return to Life Through Contrology*, and it's the first exercise that most Pilates instructors teach their students. This is no coincidence: the Hundred warms you up, stimulates your brain, gets your heart pumping and connects your mind and body.

What You Need to Know about the Hundred

The Hundred is an integral part of the warm-up to all Pilates workouts, and it warms up your body in several ways: by improving your breathing, strengthening your Powerhouse muscles, stretching and opening your spine and chest, getting your heart to pump vigorously and speeding up the circulation of blood throughout your system.

The Hundred can be an extremely challenging exercise, but beginner-level modifications make the Hundred do-able for Pilates first-timers, too. This is an important exercise to master; the core skills you learn in the Hundred are essential to the Pilates method of body conditioning (and they help keep your body operating at top form).

What Is the Hundred?

The basic Hundred movement involves lying on your back, head and shoulders lifted and curled forwards with your legs stretched up in the air at an angle determined by your current ability – the level of difficulty your body is capable of tackling safely and effectively (the lower your legs, the more strenuous the Hundred becomes). You then pump your arms up and down to stimulate your heart, while you breathe deeply. When you do the Hundred, nothing moves but your arms; your legs remain still and your stomach is scooped and powerful.

What the Hundred Does

Performing the Hundred brings you a number of important benefits:

· The Hundred improves your breathing by expanding your ribcage and lungs, especially the important and often overlooked back part of your lungs. By lengthening and strengthening the muscles that surround the ribcage, the Hundred converts your lungs into an amazing bellows for pulling new air in and pushing old air out.
· The Hundred develops a strong, flat abdomen and a solid 'core'. It works the important muscles of your Powerhouse, especially that deepest layer of your abdomen's corset muscles, the *transversus*.

- The Hundred strengthens and lengthens the spine as the top of your spine curls up and over while your legs stretch in the opposite direction.
- The Hundred focuses your mind; as the first exercise, you use it to stimulate and awaken all your Pilates principles – awareness and concentration, centring, precise control, flowing movement, oppositional energy and breathing.

The Hundred derives its name from the maximum number of arm pumping movements you do. Joseph Pilates recommended that you do not exceed ten breaths (with five pumps for each inhale and each exhale, for a total of 100 pumps) in any one exercise session, as this would put undue stress on your system.

- The Hundred stimulates your brain and nervous system by requiring you to coordinate counting, arm pumping and breathing as you maintain your body's proper form.
- The Hundred integrates your whole body into one powerful entity, as it helps connect the strength of your upper and lower body with that of your Powerhouse.

Tips and Precautions for Doing the Hundred

The Hundred is part of every workout, so it's important to get it right before you move on. Here are some pointers to keep in mind as you're learning this Pilates exercise:

- Remember that as you do the Hundred, your stomach continually draws in and up your spine (in the scoop). That means your deep breathing expands through the ribcage, into your armpits, under your collarbones and between your shoulder blades, rather than swelling your stomach outwards.
- An important part of your job in the Hundred is to strengthen your abdominals and to keep your back stable. For example, as you

exhale, imagine your stomach being pressed into and up along your spine by a powerful old-fashioned lace-up corset. Don't lose the feel of this corseted support; instead, imagine that the corset pulls tighter with each inhalation and exhalation. This way, your abdominal scoop will deepen with each breath, improving your support.

· As you do the Hundred, make sure your back remains flat and stable along the floor. Arching your back compresses the lumbar region of your spine and puts strain on your neck as well.

If you feel any straining or discomfort in your neck or lower back, adjust your position by bending or lowering your legs or broadening your shoulders and do a reduced number of repetitions. Don't continue to 'work through pain'. Your ability to perform the Hundred will improve in time.

· Keep your legs at a level that enables you to keep your back stable and along the mat. If your legs are too low during the Hundred, you put excess strain on your back and neck. If you notice that you are trying to pull up or lift away from the floor, bend your knees or raise your legs. You can lower your legs as your skills grow.

· As you curl your upper spine, shoulders and head up from the floor, your objective is to keep your shoulders wide and open so you can breathe better and free the movement of your arm from your shoulder girdle. If you notice that your shoulders have a tendency to scrunch up towards your ears or in towards your chest, release them into a broader position.

· Curl your neck and upper spine forwards together as a unit as you lengthen and stretch into the movement. Don't drag your shoulders up with your head or jut your chin out. You can strain your neck if you do the Hundred in the wrong position.

The Basic Hundred Exercise

The basic Hundred is an intermediate version of this important Pilates exercise. If you're at a beginner's level, use the beginner's modifications; later sections will present you with advanced modifications as well. No matter what your level or which modifications you use, the following steps represent the basic movement and breathing directions for this exercise.

Step by Step Through the Basic Hundred

In the Hundred, you use the Pilates scoop, Upper Body Curl and other Pilates fundamental movements discussed in Chapters 7 and 8. Here are the steps for the basic intermediate Hundred exercise:

1. Lie on your back, knees bent, feet flat on the mat, legs squeezed together. Your arms are extended along the mat, close to your sides with fingers pointing towards your feet (see FIGURE 9-1).
2. Inhale fully, scooping your stomach in and up your spine; then exhale as you curl your upper spine, shoulders and head off the floor, following the fundamental movement of the upper spinal flexion, practised in the Upper Body Curl mini-exercise (see Chapter 8). Don't

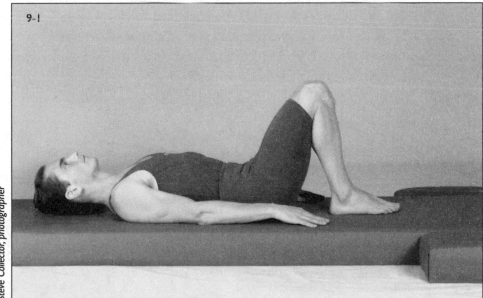

9-1

Steve Collector, photographer

just lean forwards in space; you'll crunch your abs and compress your spine. Try to coil and stretch the upper vertebrae of your spine up and over, the way a wave curls over a surfer. Ideally, the bottom tips of your shoulder blades maintain contact with the floor.

3. Allow your eyes to focus on your scooped stomach as you inhale, then exhale deeply to draw your knees up, one at a time, towards your chest while you lift your arms and hands even with your shoulder height, palms down.

   As you do the Hundred, keep your shoulders wide and your chest open. Scrunching your shoulders in towards your chest or up towards your ears inhibits your ability to breathe deeply, throws your posture out of proper alignment and ultimately diminishes the effectiveness of this exercise.

   Remember to keep your body position stable and well-supported at all times. Do this by engaging your abdominals as well as the other muscles that attach to your pelvis, including your buttocks, thighs and pelvic floor (the muscles that connect your coccyx, sitz bones and pubic bone). And don't arch your back!

4. Let your next inhale lengthen your spine in both directions; then deepen your scoop to squeeze the air out of your lungs. This action stabilizes your pelvis and lower back as you stretch your legs up and out to the angle that gives the Hundred the level of difficulty your body can safely and effectively perform. (See FIGURE 9-2A.)

5. Inhale deeply as you pump your arms in an up-and-down movement (see FIGURE 9-2B) five times; then exhale completely as you continue to

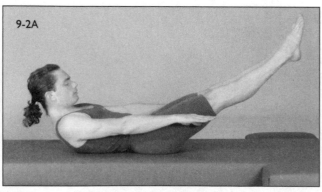

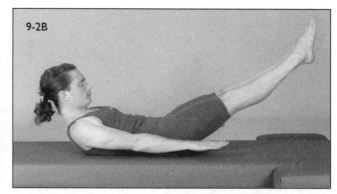

Steve Collector, photographer

pump your arms up and down another five times. Keep your wrists flat and straight, and don't lock your elbows or allow your hands or arms to touch your body or the floor. Your pumping motion should be vigorous but without strain, and should rise about 25cm (10in) off the ground.

As you pump your arms, imagine that your arms are moving against gentle resistance – as though you're pulling a canoe paddle through the water. Your arms should be strong and free of tension.

6. Repeat steps 5 and 6 up to nine times, but do not exceed 100 movements (ten complete inhalations and exhalations).

7. Keep your awareness and concentration as you slowly bend your knees to your chest, place your feet on the mat and then lower your shoulders, neck and head with control until you're at rest. Note what you feel. Are you warm? Is your stomach burning? Is your mind awake?

Things to Remember as You Do the Hundred

You get the most from the Hundred exercise if you keep some important ideas in mind as you work through the movements. Remember that each breath opens you up to further discoveries about your health, your body and your mind. Remain aware and present during the Hundred. Keep checking your body to see if you're losing your precise control. Ask yourself: is my neck relaxed? What are my shoulders doing? Are my arm-pumps smooth? Is my stomach still drawing in and up my spine? Am I exhaling as fully as I can? Are my legs still reaching long while squeezing together? In other words, keep the dialogue between your mind and your body alive.

Beginner's Modifications for the Hundred

If you're new to Pilates (and haven't been exercising regularly in any other fitness plan), you probably won't be able to accomplish a perfect version of the Hundred the first time you try it. Here are some ways to make the Hundred more approachable. As your Pilates confidence grows and your body becomes better conditioned, you will be able to slowly drop these modifications.

When you're modifying the Hundred, keep in mind the important benefits of the exercise – the warm-up, mental focusing, core strengthening, spinal stretching and lengthening, improved breathing and the integration of your whole body into one powerful entity. As you become stronger and more capable, you will automatically advance your modifications so you can continue to experience these benefits. If you make the Hundred too easy, you lose its powerful benefits, so, as with any Pilates exercise, use your judgment and continue to challenge yourself; take your progress safely and appropriately.

You can choose from three main categories of modification to make the Hundred accessible to you as a beginner. You can:

- Reduce repetitions; for example, do fifty instead of 100 pumps.
- Reduce the range of motion, by making arm pumps shallower.
- Reduce the load or effort the exercise places on important muscles and joints. For example, bend your knees (see FIGURE 9-3) to enable you to deepen your scoop. Or prop your feet on the wall so your back stays long on the mat (see FIGURE 9-4); the wall's support of your legs permits weaker abs to strengthen without back strain. Another approach would be to lift your legs higher.

You also can eliminate certain movements from the Hundred initially, then slowly add them back in as your body becomes used to the position, the breathing technique and so on.

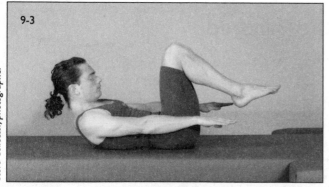

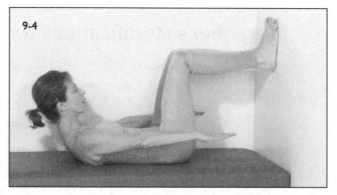

Steve Collector, photographer

Progressing Beyond the Beginner's Level

As your skills improve, you'll want to build towards the basic (and then the advanced!) Hundred exercise. To move from a complete beginner's level to a more difficult level, follow this progression:

1. The first few times you do the Hundred, lie on the mat with your knees bent, feet flat and head resting on a pillow.
2. Then begin to add movements. Start with pumping your arms as you breathe in for five pumps and out for five pumps. Focus only on your breath – inhale for five and exhale for five.
3. Next, add the upper body curl, curling your shoulders, neck and head off the floor (a fundamental skill) as you breathe in for five pumps and out for five pumps.
4. Next, fold your knees to your chest or prop your feet on a wall or a couch as you curl your shoulders, neck and head off the floor and pump your arms as you breathe – in for five pumps and out for five pumps.
5. When you're comfortable with that modification, extend your legs up to a 90-degree angle while you are curled and pumping.
6. As you begin to feel that you have no trouble holding your legs up, extended at your working-level height, slowly work on lowering them over the course of future sessions.

This progression of modifications will allow you to develop the strength and control necessary to perform the Hundred at the basic level. Your awareness of your body will increase as you become more skilled at the Hundred, and your breathing will deepen as you increase repetitions until you're able to reach the maximum of 100 per session.

The Ultimate Version of the Hundred

When you've mastered the basic version of the Hundred, you're ready to try some advanced modifications. Here are some ideas for gradually taking the Hundred to new levels:

1. Continue lowering your straight legs until they are eye height (in other words, about 38cm (15in) from the ground).
2. The next challenge is to begin the exercise lying flat on the floor with legs extended; then, on an exhale, simultaneously curl your upper body and lift your legs to eye height. Begin the arm pumps as you inhale.
3. Then, take it one step further by scissoring your legs, crossing them out and in, out and in, briskly in rhythm to your arm pumps without losing your connection to your core.
4. Squeeze a Magic Circle between your ankles to intensify the workout the Hundred gives your Powerhouse and inner thighs. (See FIGURE 9-5.)
5. Play with your breath by inhaling for sequentially fewer arm pumps while exhaling for sequentially more arm pumps; for example, in for four – out for six, in for three – out for seven, and so on.

Remember that you aren't competing with anyone but yourself. Take your modifications slowly and safely. As you build strength, flexibility and confidence, continue to challenge yourself by increasing the level of the exercise so that you continue to receive the rewards.

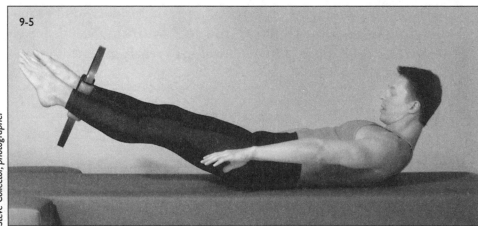

9-5

Steve Collector, photographer

Using the Hundred in Other Movements

The benefits you gain from the Hundred extend through every movement you make and everything you do. And you'll find that the skills the Hundred teaches you come in handy throughout your busy day. For example, the Hundred promotes effective breathing and powerful oxygen intake so you have an energized, focused, calm mind. The Hundred encourages you to find and strengthen your correct pelvic placement. As a result, you don't strain your lower back when you climb stairs or get out of a chair. The Hundred also develops your abdominals in order to stabilize and support your spine. That makes it easier and safer for you to vacuum, shovel snow or lift heavy objects. The Hundred aligns your shoulders and neck, so you don't suffer unnecessary pain when working with your arms raised, as when you paint your home or clean that top shelf.

Your improved range of shoulder motion will help you avoid bursitis and other painful shoulder and neck inflammations and injuries. By practising the Hundred, you build increased abdominal strength and spinal flexibility that helps you with even the most basic movements, such as rising up from your bed or getting out of the bath. Athletes find the increased breathing capacity and oxygen intake, the core stabilization

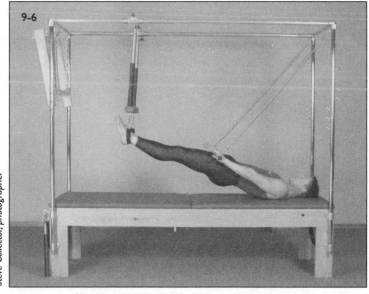

9-6

Steve Collector, photographer

and the full-body integration they gain from doing the Hundred are essential for jumping, swinging, climbing, biking and more. The ski jumper, for instance, performs the Hundred every time he or she leaves the ramp.

The skills you learn in the Hundred are so fundamental, they apply to every single exercise in the entire Pilates system – whether you're doing a headstand on the Universal Reformer or Wunda Chair, or hanging upside down off the Trapeze Table. One great example is the Breathing exercise on the Trap Table, which uses spring tension to increase the breath and the full-body integrating power of the Hundred (see FIGURE 9-6 on page 129).

'Contrology exercises build a sturdy body and sound mind, fitted to perform every daily task with ease and perfection as well as to provide tremendous reserve energy for sports, recreation, emergencies.'

Joseph Pilates, *Return to Life Through Contrology*

CHAPTER 10
The Roll-Up

The Roll-Up is essential to every Pilates mat workout. Joseph Pilates considered the action of rolling and unrolling the spine an integral part of the Pilates method. The action of rolling 'cleanses your lungs' of impurities, he said, as it 'restores your spine' to its natural state of uniform flexibility and strength. This is why so many Pilates exercises incorporate the movements and skills you learn in the Roll-Up.

What You Need to Know about the Roll-Up

The Roll-Up is an important warm-up exercise that helps limber up and stretch your joints and muscles as it gets your heart pumping and improves your breathing technique. In particular, the Roll-Up gives the joints and muscles of your spine and back a valuable 'massage' that stimulates your circulation and the portion of your nervous system housed in the spinal column. This massaging action helps the Roll-Up promote the essential mind/body connection that's such an important benefit of the Pilates method of conditioning.

The Roll-Up makes your body and mind stronger, more flexible and capable of more precise control, and it continues to expand your capabilities in these areas with each repetition. Each Roll-Up you do is slightly different from the one before as your body changes and your education and experience deepen.

Joseph Pilates devised the Roll-Up to promote deep, healthy Pilates breathing, making it an important tool for oxygenating your blood and improving your circulation, as well as to strengthen the Powerhouse muscles, and to build a strong, flexible and well-aligned spine.

What Is the Roll-Up?

The Roll-Up is similar to an old-fashioned style of sit-up, but it emphasizes stretching and articulating your spine, rather than heaving your torso off the floor. In a basic Roll-Up, you lie flat on a workout mat with your legs straight and your arms and hands extended above your eyes. In most versions of the Roll-Up, you hold a bar or rod in your hands, and with straight arms you slowly roll your spine up and forwards, one vertebra at a time, stretching your head and arms towards your toes while you maintain your scooped stomach. As you reverse, you once again scoop your abdominals in and up the front of your spine and articulate vertebra by vertebra until you return to the original position. With each repetition of the Roll-Up, your spine is more flexible and your abdominals are stronger than before.

What the Roll-Up Does

As mentioned earlier, the Roll-Up offers a number of important physical and mental benefits:

· It is a key part of any Pilates warm-up, and it's especially effective for promoting deep, healthy breathing and getting your spine and legs ready for the Pilates work ahead.
· It is also an important Pilates tool for articulating the spine and increasing its strength and flexibility.
· It gives the muscles and joints of your spine a massage, promoting increased circulation and awakening your nervous system.
· It stretches tight hamstrings and muscles in the calves, neck and armpits, while it promotes strong, flexible hip joints.
· It increases shoulder range of motion, strength and flexibility.

As with all Pilates exercises, in the Roll-Up you work to lengthen all your muscles, even as you contract them. For instance, you don't allow your abdominals to shorten, bunch or crunch as you curl forwards. Instead, you keep your abdominals long and scooped in and up along the front of your spine, even as you challenge them to lift the weight of your upper body. This action demonstrates the unique Pilates guiding principle of oppositional energy, and it's an essential technique for developing powerful, supple muscle tissue and building a strong and flexible body.

You will feel the impact of the preceding benefits immediately, but the Roll-Up also has some long-range benefits that make themselves apparent over a period of time. Among these are:

· Long, healthy hamstrings (the muscles that run up the back of your thighs): strong and flexible hamstrings are essential to a healthy spine and proper pelvic alignment. If your hamstrings are short, stiff and tight, they hold the pelvis rigid and compromise the movement of your legs and spine; in time, these posture and movement problems can result in hip, knee, lower-back, shoulder, and neck problems.

·   A well-developed shoulder girdle: regular practice of the Roll-Up releases neck and shoulder tension, promoting healthy movement and an erect, stable posture. A healthy shoulder girdle and well-aligned posture help you breathe deeply and think clearly.

·   The long-term benefits of a strong, flexible spine and powerful abdominals, all of which promote a pain-free and injury-free life.

Tips and Precautions for Doing the Roll-Up

The Roll-Up is a safe, effective exercise, but you do need to keep a few things in mind as you're learning the proper Roll-Up technique:

·   Be sure to use your stomach muscles (scooping them in and up along the front of your spine) to lift your head, spine and arms up and over towards your feet; do *not* overuse your back.

·   Keep your arms and wrists straight but not locked as you reach forwards with them. This will help alleviate any strain on your shoulders and neck.

·   Make your movements sequential and smooth, yet strong. Don't heave your torso up. You may find that one area of your spine is less flexible than the rest. To keep your Roll-Up smooth and flowing, try timing your exhalation at different points in the Roll-Up to give your abdominal muscles more uniform strength as you lift the less-flexible portion of your spine from the floor. If you exhale at the most difficult moment of your curl, you can gain more articulation there.

·   Tight muscles need to be coaxed and massaged, not strained and pulled. Use the exercise to stretch your back and hamstrings gently in time. You aren't competing with anyone to see how far you can stretch towards your toes.

·   Remember to reach forwards with your head and spine as well as your hands. Don't strain your neck or shoulders.

· Keep your legs squeezed together and straight, reaching down along the mat; anchor your feet under a foot strap or a piece of furniture if necessary.
· Keep your pelvis stable. Don't allow your pelvis to tuck under or arch up as you lift your upper body.
· Above all, keep breathing!

The Basic Roll-Up Exercise

The steps in the following section outline the standard procedure for performing the Roll-Up at an intermediate level. Later sections offer modifications for beginners and advanced-level students of Pilates. Whatever your current skill and fitness level, you can adapt the following exercise by applying the appropriate modifications to these basic steps.

Step by Step Through the Basic Roll-Up

To transition from the Hundred, inhale as you lengthen your legs down along the mat while squeezing them together and flexing your feet up. If you're using a bar, pick it up and hold it with your hands shoulder-width apart.

In this position, exhale as you lift your arms towards the ceiling (see FIGURE 10-1), then follow these steps:

1. Inhale as you curl your head, neck and shoulders off the ground sequentially and smoothly, until your head is between your arms

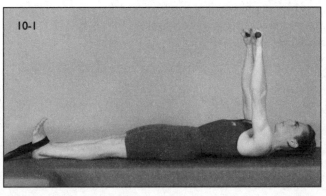
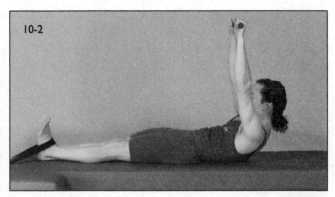

Steve Collector, photographer

(see FIGURE 10-2). Continue to roll up vertebra by vertebra until your ribcage is off the mat.

2. Exhaling, scoop your stomach deeper in and up along the front of your spine as you continue to articulate your vertebrae (exactly as a wheel) until you've curled your whole torso off the mat and your head and hands are reaching for your feet. (See FIGURES 10-3 and 10-4.) Your spine and arms are now parallel to the floor and your head is still trying to stay between your arms. Remember to keep the muscles around your pelvis actively engaged and your knees straight and squeezed together. At this point every muscle in your body is stretching or working and the movement of rolling forward has pushed all the air out of your lungs.

3. Inhale as you begin rolling your pelvis and then your spine back to the mat. Remember that breathing in draws your stomach in and up along your spine and away from your hamstrings and inner thighs as they reach down along the mat towards your feet – an important source of oppositional energy. Gently lay (do not press) one vertebra at a time back along the mat, scooping your stomach and elongating your spine.

4. Exhaling, continue to unroll backwards until you've sequentially stretched out your entire spine, shoulders, neck and head on the mat. Your arms are above your eyes reaching for the ceiling, as you resume the position you had at the beginning of the Roll-Up.

5. Repeat steps 1 to 4, five to eight times. With each repetition of the exercise, try to increase the length and depth of your stretch, the degree of articulation in your spine and the fullness of your inhale and your exhale.

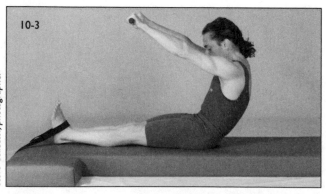
10-3

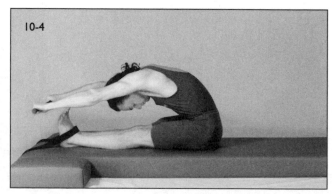
10-4

Steve Collector, photographer

Things to Remember as You Do the Roll-Up

As you work through the Roll-Up, you quickly discover it's an exercise that only looks simple. In fact, the Roll-Up requires close concentration, good muscle control and lots of flexibility. Expect to get better at this exercise with practice; to make the best progress with the Roll-Up, remember these points:

- Keep your legs and feet still as you roll and unroll your spine like a curling wave. Don't let your legs be pulled back into the wave's undertow; reach them down along the mat in opposition to your spine's movement to stabilize them.
- Remember to squeeze your legs tightly together, keeping your feet flexed and your ankles touching. This action also helps to stabilize your lower body as your upper body moves through the exercise.
- Instead of envisioning that only your hands are reaching towards your feet, reach with your spine and head, too; don't hunch your shoulders or crane your neck.

If you feel neck, shoulder, or lower-back strain during the Roll-Up, stop and determine what's causing it. If your position and breathing technique seem to be right, try one or more modifications listed in this chapter to find a version of the Roll-Up that works for you now. Challenge your body with Pilates, but do it safely.

- When rolling and unrolling in the Roll-Up, use a few visualization techniques to articulate your spine correctly. Imagine you're doing the exercise on a cloud, for example, and you can't press down too hard with your spine or pelvis or you'll fall through. Imagine your spine unrolls in the same way a rolled-up party tooter does when you blow into it. This will help develop uniform spinal articulation. Or imagine that the ceiling is very low, and you must bend under it as you roll and unroll your spine.
- Don't forget to inhale and exhale fully during the Roll-Up and to maintain full-body awareness during the entire exercise. Deep

breathing and strong concentration and awareness are two of your biggest allies in learning and gaining maximum benefit from the Roll-Up exercise.

Beginner's Modifications for the Roll-Up

Even the basic intermediate version of the Roll-Up is extremely demanding, so don't expect to whizz through it the first time you try. If the basic Roll-Up is beyond your current skill level, don't be discouraged. You can get started on the road to mastering this exercise by applying one or more beginner-level modifications. These modifications are designed to help you reap the benefits of the exercise – a strong, healthy, flexible, well-aligned spine, a powerful, supple core and deep, healthy breathing – safely at your current skill level. As your body becomes stronger and more flexible, you will use fewer beginner's modifications to slowly increase the challenges of the Roll-Up so you can continue to experience its benefits.

As you modify the Roll-Up, make sure the exercise remains consistent with your current working level and your ability to perform the exercise safely and effectively. Each of your first modifications should help advance you towards the goal of developing a deeper capability and understanding of the Roll-Up.

Here's a modification of the Roll-Up that works well for many novice Pilates students. This modification works well if tight hamstrings, weak abdominals or an inflexible spine prevent you from doing the basic Roll-Up; as your strength and flexibility increase, allow your movement to go further. Here's what you do:

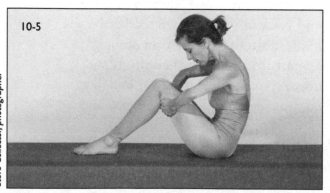

10-5

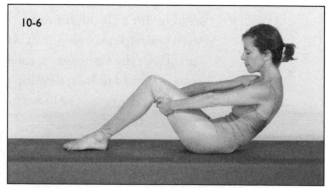

10-6

Steve Collector, photographer

1. Start the Roll-Up from a sitting position, legs together, knees bent and feet flat.
2. Grasp your thighs just below your knees, and bend your spine as much as you can to curl the top of your head towards your knees (see FIGURE 10-5).
3. Inhale slowly and scoop your stomach as you roll your spine backwards towards the mat, vertebra by vertebra; don't move your hands. When your arms are straight, stop unrolling (see FIGURE 10-6).
4. Exhale as you curl your spine back up towards your knees, one vertebra at a time; bend your elbows wide as you pull your stomach in and up along the front of your spine. Try to curl your spine even more than before as you round forwards to the starting position.
5. Repeat steps 1 to 4, five to eight times.

When doing the Roll-Up from a sitting position, it's important to keep your stomach scooped in and up. To help keep the proper position, pretend you have a hedgehog on your lap and you have to bend forwards and over it without letting it prick you!

Progressing Beyond the Beginner's Level

As your skill with the Roll-Up grows, you can increase the difficulty of the exercise to slowly advance towards the basic intermediate version. Here are a few suggestions:

· As you roll your spine back towards the mat in step 4 of the beginner's modification of the Roll-Up, let your hands slide down your thighs and continue rolling back to place your spine, one vertebra at a time, flat on the mat. As you roll up, reach for your thighs and walk your hands up your thighs towards your knees.

To progress through more difficult beginner modifications of the Roll-Up, remember to squeeze out every atom of air during your exhalation, so you keep strengthening your stomach and stretching your back.

- Try rolling down and up without using your hands at all.
- With each repetition, move your feet further away from your hips, allowing your arms to slide along the mat at your sides.
- When you're able to start the Roll-Up by lying flat, with your legs straight and squeezed together and your feet fully flexed, pick up the bar and advance to the basic intermediate Roll-Up version.

The Ultimate Version of the Roll-Up

When you've mastered the basic intermediate version of the Roll-Up, you're ready to try some advanced modifications. Here are some ideas for taking the Roll-Up to new levels:

1. Gradually lower the starting position of the bar and arms until you can lay them flat on the mat above your head. Keep your shoulders wide and flat, and don't allow your ribcage to arch off the mat. (If necessary, review the Ribcage Arms mini-exercise in Chapter 8.)
2. Next, begin the Roll-Up by raising your arms until they are perpendicular to the floor, curl your head and shoulders off the mat until your head is between your arms, and then continue to roll up and down. Keep your head between your arms the entire time until your arms are again perpendicular to the floor. To finish, lower your shoulders and head, then reach your arms back to the mat above your head.
3. Finally, curl your head, shoulders and arms simultaneously. Keep your arms next to your head throughout the entire exercise, but (especially at the beginning and end) remember that your shoulders must remain relaxed down away from your ears *and* you still have to articulate one vertebra at a time! Keep your legs firmly anchored together and reaching down along the mat.

Using the Roll-Up in Other Movements

You're as old as your spine is flexible! By lengthening your spine and abdominals in the Roll-Up, you provide more room for your organs and lungs, and you stand taller and breathe better. The Roll-Up also teaches you the very important skill of distinguishing your arm movement from your shoulder movement. Bursitis, tendonitis, frozen shoulder and rotator cuff injuries can all stem from improper shoulder girdle and joint mechanics. A strong, flexible shoulder girdle and joint enable you to safely reach, stretch and lift without strain or pain. Tight, stiff or over-bulky hamstrings inhibit good spinal and pelvic movement patterns. The Roll-Up lengthens and balances these powerful cables so your whole body moves with more efficiency and ease. As you become more flexible and resilient, the movements of your hip joints, pelvis and spine become stronger and more fluid – which, in turn, helps you to avoid injuries that result from bad posture and repetitive movement.

The skills you develop in the Roll-Up help you in a wide variety of physical activities. Your increased abdominal power, spine flexibility, precision of hip movement and overall muscle resiliency will enable you to lift and move objects without straining your back. And bending tasks, such as raking leaves, vacuuming or shovelling snow from the drive, won't take such a strong toll on your lower back. As your spine and abdominals grow stronger, you'll find that you can stand longer without tiring (which comes in very handy at the airport or at trade shows).

If you practise sports, the Roll-Up benefits your technique in a number of ways. Your improved shoulder range of motion and strength will help you in any athletic movement that requires your arms to reach high or far from your body, such as serving a tennis ball or volleyball. With improved stability and agility you can access your core power to enable more efficient and effective swings in games such as tennis, volleyball and golf. By uniformly developing all your muscles, the Roll-Up enhances your endurance for activities such as cycling, cross-country skiing, swimming and diving. Rock climbers find that the increased shoulder and hamstring flexibility gives them the range to reach further for holds and the ability to climb more difficult routes without injury.

In Pilates, the Roll-Up prepares your mind and body for more advanced exercises, such as the Tendon Stretch on the Universal Reformer, and Inversions and Monkey on the Trapeze Table. The Upside-Down Push-Up on the Low Chair takes all the skills you learn in the Roll-

Up – shoulder integration, abdominal strength, spinal flexibility, and more – to a whole new level (SEE FIGURE 10-7).

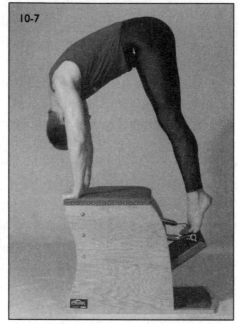

Steve Collector, photographer

'If your spine is inflexibly stiff at 30, you are old; if it's completely flexible at 60, you are young... the only real guide to your true age lies not in years, or how old you THINK you feel, but... by the degree of natural and normal flexibility enjoyed by your spine throughout life.'

Joseph Pilates, letter to clients, 1939

CHAPTER 11

The Single Leg Circle

The Single Leg Circle continues to warm up your body, expand your breathing capacity, focus your mind and strengthen your centre, but it takes your warm-up one important step further by limbering up your hip joints in a bigger range of motion. Here's where you really begin to train your hip joints to move precisely, correctly and healthily.

What You Need to Know
about the Single Leg Circle

The Single Leg Circle is the first asymmetrical mat-work exercise you learn in this series; in this exercise, your legs do two different things simultaneously. This asymmetrical way of moving challenges your mind, your nervous system, your stability, your coordination and your whole-body awareness. It also reveals asymmetries – or imbalances – in your body's skeletal and muscular structure. At the same time, this exercise engages both legs as they support and are being supported by the rest of the body. Overall, the Single Leg Circle requires (and develops) more precise control and muscular balance.

Don't be surprised if you discover that you can do this exercise more easily with one leg than with the other. This 'side dominance' is typical for most people and results from a lack of uniform development. As you gain skill with the Single Leg Circle and other Pilates exercises, you will see these differences diminish.

What Is the Single Leg Circle?

When performing the Single Leg Circle, you lie flat on your back, arms extended along the mat close to your sides, with one leg stretched straight along the mat and the other leg reaching up to the ceiling at a 90-degree angle from your pelvis. Keeping both legs long and both feet softly pointed, you move your raised leg to describe a circle about the size of a hula hoop in the air over your other leg. After a set number of circles, you reverse direction; then you switch legs and repeat the circles.

One of your biggest challenges in performing the Single Leg Circle is to keep your bottom leg, spine, head, arms and palms anchored along the mat while your raised leg performs precise, controlled movements. The oppositional energy required to support these two distinct actions makes the Single Leg Circle a powerful Pilates exercise.

What the Single Leg Circle Does

This exercise really shines in its ability to teach you to stabilize, anchor and move various parts of your body in different ways simultaneously; to develop intense core strength; and to promote deep healthy breathing and strong circulation. The Single Leg Circle is a fantastic way to reveal imbalances in your hip joints and hamstrings. Short, stiff hamstrings prevent you from accessing full pelvic range of motion and stability, something that is vitally important to your overall physical health. The more you know about your particular restrictions and capabilities, the better able you are to make the Single Leg Circle – and all Pilates exercises – more effective for you. Following are some other benefits of this wonderful exercise:

- Improved range and efficiency of movement in your hip joints.
- Strong legs and hips, and a stronger, more stable lower back and spine.
- Balanced muscular use and strength of legs, hips, shoulders and torso, to help avoid arthritis, tendonitis and general degeneration of the hip and knee joints.
- A longer, stronger spine, resulting from Pilates' unique way of building both power and length simultaneously.

Imbalances in the way you stand and walk are big contributors to weak, painful hip joints – a common problem for the elderly. The Single Leg Circle works in conjunction with other Pilates exercises to promote uniformly developed muscle and joint strength, and to eliminate the chronic wear and tear these imbalances place on our body's structure.

Tips and Precautions for Doing the Single Leg Circle

The Single Leg Circle offers a wide variety of benefits, as long as you do it correctly. Otherwise, you not only limit the benefits you gain from the exercise, but you might even strain certain muscles. Follow these general guidelines to keep the Single Leg Circle effective and healthy:

· Coordinated breathing is a must for all Pilates exercises, and the Single Leg Circle is no exception. As you lengthen your leg, air is pulled into your lungs, and as you circle the leg and return it to the centre, the movement helps your abdominals squeeze the air from your lungs.

· Keep your pelvis level and stable. Don't allow your pelvis to tuck under or rotate sideways as you extend your leg up into the air. These tendencies result from tight hamstring, inner-thigh, lower-back or hip muscles.

· Use oppositional energy to elongate your whole body, so it feels like a spring being stretched between your feet and head. This image gives you better access to your core strength and helps you avoid overusing your neck, shoulders and lower back. At the same time, keep your shoulders wide; don't allow them to scrunch up while you raise and circle your leg.

Many Pilates students find that placing a small pillow under their head during this exercise helps them maintain good shoulder and neck alignment. If you use a pillow, make sure it's no more than a few centimetres thick and rests only under your head and neck, not under your shoulders.

· When you make the circles with your leg (especially as you lower the leg away from you), always focus on your scoop (review this fundamental Pilates skill in Chapters 7 and 8). Scooping your stomach in and up along your spine stabilizes your torso and keeps your back from arching.

· Don't let your foot swing more than a few centimetres out, past the outside of your hip, when you're making the circles. Doing so can put dangerous strains on your groin muscles and may pull the opposite hip off the mat, which could put stress on your lower back. Be even more aware of this important safety issue when circling your leg in the second direction.

Use the beginner-level modifications if you find that you struggle to follow any one of these guidelines or if you feel any pain or strain while performing the Single Leg Circle. As your skills grow, you can evolve your modifications until you're capable of doing the basic intermediate version. Then you can move on towards the more advanced versions listed at the end of this chapter.

The Basic Single Leg Circle Exercise

The following section outlines the steps for performing the Single Leg Circle at an intermediate level. Following the presentation of these steps, you'll find modifications for beginners and advanced-level students of Pilates.

Step by Step Through the Basic Single Leg Circle

To transition from the Roll-Up, inhale as you fold your right knee to your chest; and exhale as you place both your hands on your right shin. Squeeze your leg to you to stretch and release any tension in that hip (this action frees up the motion of your hip and leg), then follow these steps:

1. Inhale as you extend your right leg straight up, at a 90-degree angle from your pelvis. Place both hands behind your right thigh and exhale as you gently pull your leg towards you three times, then return your

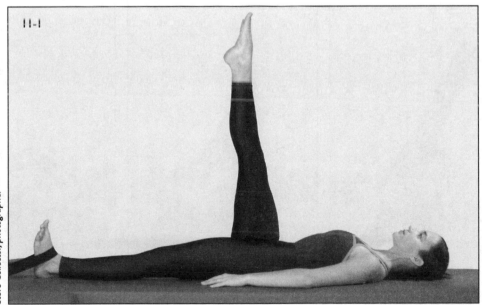

11-1

Steve Collector, photographer

arms to your side, and leave your raised leg in its 90-degree position (see FIGURE 11-1). Stretch both your legs away from your pelvis as your stomach scoops in and up along the front of your spine in preparation for the Single Leg Circle.

2. Inhale as you draw your stomach in and up along the front of your spine and circle your right leg across your body and down towards your left foot, continuing halfway around the circle (see FIGURES 11-2 and 11-3). Keep your pelvis, spine, neck and arms anchored along the floor as you circle your leg over your body. Remember to maintain length in all your muscles even as you contract them!

3. Exhale powerfully to squeeze all the air out of your lungs and deepen your scoop; this action pulls your leg up and through the second half of the circle (see FIGURE 11-4), where it returns to the starting position.

Repeat steps 2 and 3 of the Single Leg Circle four more times; then reverse the direction of your circles, and perform the Single Leg Circle five times.

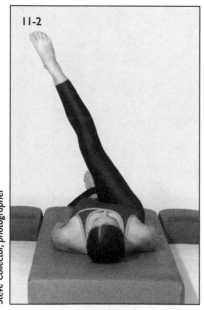

11-2

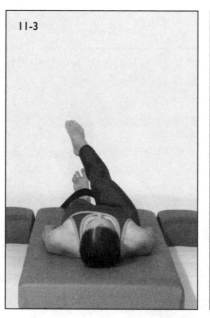

11-3

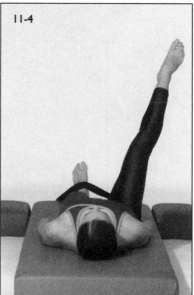

11-4

Steve Collector, photographer

Note that just as your deep exhalation helps pull your leg up in the Single Leg Circle, the upward movement of your leg conversely helps deepen your exhalation and more completely empty your lungs of air. This coordination of movement and breath is used throughout Pilates to deepen your breathing and improve your core strength.

Another point to keep in mind: as you circle your raised leg, keep reaching your opposite leg down along the mat. Don't allow it to shorten or bend. Stretch your raised leg away from you as you lengthen both hips away from your ribs to keep your pelvis and spine positions stable and your abdominals long and scooped.

To continue with the other leg, follow these steps:

1. Inhale as you bend your right knee to your chest, squeeze it in with both hands, then exhale deeply as you lower your right leg down along the mat beside the left one.
2. Bend your left knee in to you and repeat the entire process, using your left leg. When you've completed ten circles with your left leg (five in each direction), inhale to bend your left knee to your shoulder and exhale to give it a squeeze with both hands.

With each circle your leg describes in the Single Leg Circle, you will notice that you have increased flexibility, strength and precision in your movement. To maximize this movement-by-movement gain, ask yourself: 'What more can I get from each repetition?'

Things to Remember as You Do the Single Leg Circle

It's not easy to circle one leg in a precise, controlled movement while you keep the rest of your body stable and anchored to the mat. Don't become discouraged if it takes a while for you to get this exercise under your belt; you'll get better at it with practice. Meanwhile, keep these points in mind to get the most from the Single Leg Circle:

· Make precise circles with your leg.
· Keep searching your body with your mind to check your Pilates breathing, pelvic and ribcage stability, scoop and your use of oppositional energy.

- Make your breath an integral and coordinated part of the movement.
- Keep your stomach scooped in and up along the front of your elongated spine as you stabilize your pelvis.
- Keep your shoulders broad and your arms close to your sides and pressed down along the mat; this position helps prevent your torso from rocking as your leg circles.
- Alternate the leg you start with from session to session to promote uniform development.
- To develop precise and powerful range of motion in your hip, pretend you're drawing a circle on the ceiling with the toes of your raised foot.
- Use oppositional energy to reach your legs apart from one another; this in turn centres you as it decompresses your lower back and hip joints.
- Keep your kneecaps pointing straight forwards – don't allow your legs to turn in or out.

Finally, remember not to let your leg open too far to the outside of your body as you move it in a circle. You'll know when you've gone too far because you won't be able to keep your pelvis from tilting sideways.

Beginner's Modifications for the Single Leg Circle

The Single Leg Circle can be challenging to anyone with tight hamstrings or weak abdominals or lower-back muscles – and those are the people who need this exercise most. Don't be discouraged if you aren't ready to leap right into the basic intermediate version; this exercise can be modified in a number of ways to make it more approachable for anyone, yet still challenging enough to advance you towards more proficiency. Use any (or all) of the modifications listed in this section of the chapter (but only for as long as you need to).

Your First Modifications

As with any Pilates exercise, your most important consideration when modifying the Single Leg Circle is to make sure you're getting the maximum benefit from the exercise, rather than trying to match your version to some predefined beginner or advanced level. Here are some modifications that work well for many students:

· If you can't straighten your raised leg all the way, bend it as much as necessary to maintain pelvic and spine stability as you circle the leg.
· You can also try bending the bottom leg instead of the raised leg, but again, only as much as necessary to help you remain stable and still benefit from the effect of oppositional energy.
· If you need to further reduce the pull of your hamstrings and hip muscles, bend both knees, but again, only as much as is necessary to do the leg circles without tucking or tilting your pelvis.
· Draw smaller circles with your raised foot.
· Reduce the number of circles you make in each phase of the exercise.

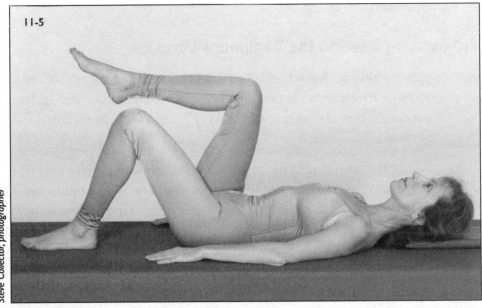

11-5

Steve Collector, photographer

Here's a stepped procedure for a beginner's modification of the Single Leg Circle:

1. Lie on the mat, a small pillow under your head, knees bent, feet flat and arms by your sides. Breathe calmly and evenly.
2. Raise one foot to bring your shin parallel to the floor (see FIGURE 11-5). This beginner's modification makes the Single Leg Circle do-able, yet it is still challenging for anyone with tight hamstrings or an unstable pelvis.
3. Continuing your breathing, imagine that your kneecap is a pencil or paintbrush and draw a small circle – the size of a 10 pence coin – on an imaginary piece of paper suspended a couple of centimetres above your knee.
4. Repeat the circle five to ten times, then reverse.
5. Switch legs, and repeat steps 1 through 4.

When you perform this modification of the Single Leg Circle, focus on the feeling of your femur (thigh bone) moving precisely in your hip socket while you scoop your stomach in to keep your pelvis stable. Keep the Pilates guiding principles in mind: concentration and awareness, Pilates breathing, centring, precise control, flowing movement and oppositional energy.

Progressing Beyond the Beginner's Level

As your skill with the Single Leg Circle builds, you can adjust your modifications to move towards the basic intermediate, then more advanced versions. Here are some ideas for working towards the full intermediate version of this exercise:

· As the movement in your hip becomes more precise and fluid, begin straightening one or the other of your legs – you may want to experiment to see which leg to straighten first. When you straighten your upper leg you may find that a tight hamstring makes you struggle to keep your pelvis neutral, not tucked. But when you straighten the bottom leg you may find that your stomach isn't quite strong enough to keep your back from arching. Which modification serves you better? Learning the answer to this question will help you progress.

· Get your Pilates teacher or workout partner to hold your ankle down (to help you stabilize your core more effectively), until you no longer need this support (see FIGURE 11-6). Keep elongating your leg away from your centre.

· If you're straightening the bottom leg all the way, you may find it easier to put that foot under the edge of a couch or chair to help keep it stable.

· When you're able to straighten both legs while still maintaining a stable Powerhouse, spine and pelvis, start making larger circles.

· Increase the number of circles, until you're capable of doing the basic intermediate version's limit of five circles, 1.2m (4 ft) in diameter, in each phase of the exercise while still maintaining an elongated spine, stable shoulders and pelvis, and straight legs.

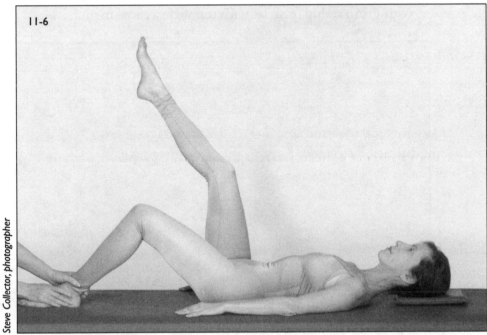

11-6

Steve Collector, photographer

The Ultimate Version of the Single Leg Circle

When you've mastered the basic intermediate version of the Single Leg Circle you're ready to try some advanced modifications. Here are some ideas:

·   Make even larger circles (but only if you can maintain precise control, straight legs and a stable pelvis and spine).

·   Begin your circle by reaching your toes towards your opposite ear (see FIGURE 11-7). Keep your hip reaching in opposition to your toes, but allow it to be stretched and lengthened off the mat by this movement. Your spine will be pulled into a small twist. This twisting action stimulates the nervous system housed in your spine; stretches your lower back, buttocks and outer hip and thigh; and further strengthens your abdominal muscles and inner thighs.

Continue drawing a large circle with your toes that reaches all the way down to your other foot and then opens a little wider to the outside as it completes its path. Don't go too far to the outside, though! Even though you're capable of moving further out than you were when you did the basic intermediate version, you still need to beware of straining your groin or hip muscles with too wide a movement.

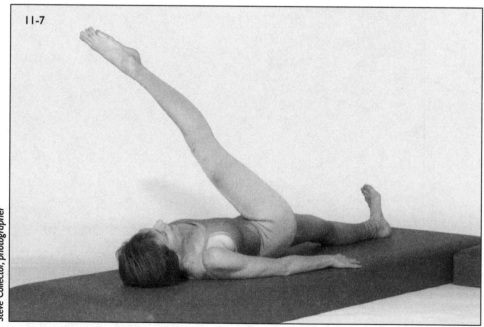

11-7

Steve Collector, photographer

Using the Single Leg Circle in Other Movements

Strong hips, legs, spine and abdominal muscles benefit you in almost anything you do during a busy, active day. Healthy hips will keep you running and walking, standing, climbing stairs, bending and lifting with much greater ease – and no pain! The Single Leg Circle also builds strong abdominal muscles, which support your spine to eliminate lower-back strain and keep you looking fit and trim. Every time you sweep your floor, shovel snow, rake leaves or get in or out of your car, your body will benefit from the workout it received from the Single Leg Circle.

Athletes and sports enthusiasts love the benefits they get from the Single Leg Circle. Many sports, including skiing, skating, cycling, tennis, golf and cricket, depend on the strength, stability and flexibility this exercise promotes in the Powerhouse, legs and spine. More resilient hips, lower back and spine help with speed, endurance and agility, and protect against the forces that impact your body as you play sports – for example, the jolts you get each time you land on your feet during running.

As you move into more advanced Pilates work, you'll use the skills you build in this exercise to do such movements as Hanging Down with a Twist on the Trapeze Table, Twist I on the Mat and Tree with Arch on the High Barrel (see FIGURE 11-8), an exercise in which you perform an

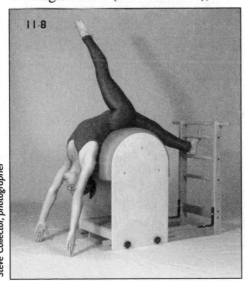

11-8

Steve Collector, photographer

extremely advanced version of the Single Leg Circle, upside down with a fully arched spine, both arms reaching beyond the head, and the whole position supported only by the connection at one ankle. All of these added challenges promote more uniform development, flexible and decompressed spine and joints, and a powerful body/mind/spirit connection. The exercise also promotes an internal shower and deep Pilates breathing.

'A body freed from... over-fatigue is the ideal shelter provided by nature for housing a well-balanced mind that is always capable of successfully meeting all the complex problems of modern living.'

Joseph Pilates, *Return to Life Through Contrology*

CHAPTER 12

Rolling
Like a Ball

The Rolling Like a Ball exercise is unique to the Pilates method of body conditioning, and it's a definitive exercise in the system. This movement is designed to help you breathe deeply and fully and to restore the spine to its healthy, elongated, natural alignment – two of the primary Pilates goals.

What You Need to Know about Rolling Like a Ball

This quintessential exercise stretches and massages your entire spine, strengthens your core and helps you breathe deeply. As you move through the mat-work series, notice that the order of the exercises requires you to change positions frequently, keeping your entire body active and moving – flexing, stretching, twisting, turning over, sitting up, lying on your back, then on your stomach, then your side – just as you do in life.

Joseph Pilates purposefully designed the mat-work series to support and strengthen natural human movements. For instance, when you do the Single Leg Circle, you keep your spine straight and stable throughout the exercise. Consequently, this follow-up exercise requires you to flex and roll your spine, so your muscles continue to grow stronger and more flexible without tightening or bulking up.

As part of your warm-up, you work your body in these first Pilates exercises in much the same way a baker kneads bread dough. By flexing, stretching and warming your muscles, expanding your breathing and boosting your circulation, you prepare your body for all of the action that lies ahead – both in the Pilates studio and in your daily activities.

What Is Rolling Like a Ball?

Performing the basic Rolling Like a Ball movement involves sitting up, bending your knees to your chest, holding your lower shins with both hands and curling your spine and head up and over your knees until you feel round like a ball. In this position, you roll backwards and forwards, up and down your spine, in order to massage your back on the mat. As you roll, your spine is fully curled and your eyes are focused on your stomach.

What the Rolling Like a Ball Exercise Does

Rolling Like a Ball is a great exercise for articulating and strengthening your spine, but its benefits go well beyond that important function. This exercise is an excellent way to develop deep, healthy Pilates breathing. As you roll back, the movement pulls air into your lungs, causing your back to inflate and your vertebrae and ribcage to expand and decompress. Your forward-rolling movement pushes the air from your lungs in a deep, healthy exhalation. Each repetition strengthens your stomach as you squeeze your abdominals to push the air from your lungs. The massaging action of the rolling encourages healthy circulation as it elongates the muscles in your back, hips and shoulders. Here are some other benefits of this amazing exercise:

· A stronger integration between your Powerhouse and pelvis (gluteals, pelvic floor, inner thighs, hamstrings and back muscles).
· Better shoulder girdle stabilization and integration skills.
· Improved balance and coordination.
· Better full-body integration to facilitate a mind/body connection.

Rolling Like a Ball draws heavily on the Pilates principles of precise control and concentration and awareness. You must maintain precise control of your body's position and movement, even in a disorienting, upside-down position. Your ability to concentrate and be actively aware of your movements helps you do several complex tasks simultaneously – all of which is great Pilates practice.

Tips and Precautions for the Rolling Like a Ball Exercise

Rolling Like a Ball can be a very difficult exercise. When you're learning and practising this exercise, you need to keep several important guidelines in mind in order to get the most benefit from it.

Here are some important tips and precautions:

· Stop the backward roll when you reach the area between your shoulder blades. Your head and neck never touch the mat.
· Make your rolling motion smooth and sequential; if you find yourself flopping or crashing backwards like a flat tyre instead of a round

wheel, use modifications offered later in this chapter to maintain smooth, flowing motion.

- Keep your eyes focused on your stomach throughout the exercise. Don't throw your head around to create momentum for the rolling motion.
- To promote a full, healthy lower-spine curl, visualize that you're reaching your sitz bones or coccyx towards the back of your knees as you scoop your stomach in and up. This visualization uses the guiding principle of oppositional energy to strengthen your gluteals and hamstrings and to stretch lower-back tightness.

The old saying, 'when in doubt, leave it out', definitely applies to this exercise. Don't attempt it if you have any of the following issues: osteoporosis, herniated or bulging vertebral discs, rods in your spine, current or recent cervical injuries, severe scoliosis or spondylolisthesis, among others. Be safe, and get your doctor's approval before attempting this exercise.

- Imagine that you're squeezing a ball between your knees while you roll back and forth. This squeezing motion helps you access the power of your belly, inner thighs and pelvic muscles as it stretches out your lower back.
- When you curl your upper spine, keep your shoulders open and broad, with your shoulder blades reaching down your back and your elbows lifted and wide. Don't allow your shoulders to scrunch up towards your ears or forwards into your chest.
- Visualize your spine-curling motion as that of a poster being rolled up to fit into a mailing tube. Curl your spine over at the top, vertebra by vertebra, rather than folding your shoulders in upon themselves or crunching your abdominals. Each end of your spine curls away from the other with balanced, oppositional energy.
- Roll evenly down the middle of your spine, as if you were rolling along a channel or a railroad track. Your natural tendency may be to roll towards one side of your spine, so pay careful attention and correct any side preferences you see cropping up.

The Basic Rolling Like a Ball Exercise

The steps in the following section outline the basic procedure for performing the Rolling Like a Ball exercise at an intermediate level. Again, this exercise can be very difficult, and many people find the backward-rolling movement a bit disorienting, so take your time and play with the exercise to get comfortable with it. And never fear – this exercise can be modified in a number of ways. You'll find modifications for beginners and advanced Pilates students following the basic steps.

Step by Step Through the Basic Exercise

To transition from the Single Leg Circle, inhale to bend your left knee and squeeze it into your chest with both hands, then, as you exhale, keep both hands on your left shin and curl your head, shoulders and upper body forwards as you roll your spine up off the mat, vertebra by vertebra, to a sitting position. Inhale as you bend your right knee into your chest and hold both lower shins; your knees are shoulder-width apart, your heels are touching, and your elbows are high and wide. Exhale to curl your spine even more, pulling your stomach deep into and up along the front of your

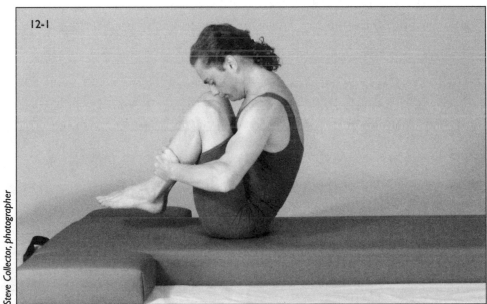

12-1

Steve Collector, photographer

spine as you curl your head between your knees, eyes on your stomach. Imagine that your stomach is massaging your internal organs and spine. Carefully rock back onto your coccyx just far enough to balance; your softly pointed toes should be hovering slightly above the mat (see FIGURE 12-1). Now, follow these steps to perform the basic intermediate Rolling Like a Ball exercise:

1. Inhale, letting your breath lengthen your spine up and over like a wave curling over a surfer, as you curl your tail under you and roll your spine backwards, one vertebra at a time (see FIGURE 12-2); roll with a smooth, flowing motion down the mat, until you're on your spine between your shoulder blades (see FIGURE 12-3). Suspend your hips as high above you as you can without rolling onto your neck.
2. Exhale to roll back down your spine, returning to your original balancing position on your coccyx with your toes just off the mat. As you roll forwards, use your arms to pull your legs in to you to further strengthen and challenge your stomach and to help you exhale. Keep elbows lifted and wide.
3. Repeat steps 1 and 2, five to eight times.

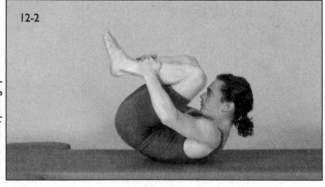

12-2

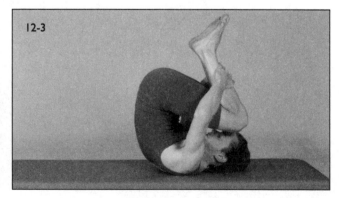

12-3

Steve Collector, photographer

If you feel any strain or discomfort in your neck, mid-back or lower back during Rolling Like a Ball, stop and assess your movements. Perhaps you're rolling up too far, putting pressure on your head or neck. Or perhaps you need to modify the exercise to make it more accessible for your current condition. Modify as necessary, but don't work through the pain!

Things to Remember as You Perform This Exercise

Rolling Like a Ball may look like a child's recreation, but it can challenge even the most seasoned Pilates student. You'll get better over time, but when you're first starting out with this incredible exercise, keep these points in mind for best results:

- With each succeeding repetition of the Rolling Like a Ball movement, your muscles become more responsive, joints become more flexible and so on. So each time you repeat the rolling movement, increase your awareness of your body and its increasing capabilities. Continually work to improve your centring, breathing, flowing motion, pelvic and shoulder stability and balance.

Do I need a special mat for the Rolling Like a Ball exercise?
A dense foam mat, such as a closed-cell camping mat or thick exercise mat, gives ample spine protection. If your spine is particularly bony, you may need an extra-thick workout mat. Don't try this exercise on any mat that's thin (like a yoga mat) or damaged, because it won't give your spine adequate protection, and you could bruise your vertebrae as your roll.

- Visualization is an important key to finding and maintaining the proper position as you roll in this exercise. Using the principle of oppositional energy, imagine that your sitz bones (or even hamstrings) and head are reaching in opposite directions towards your knees. Or imagine that you're stretching the top of your head up and over your knees like a fountain of water cascading while your sitz bones reach for the backs of your knees or even beyond your knees to the top of your head where they meet that cascading fountain. Scoop your stomach in and up the front of your spine as you do this.

· When you return to the starting position, you may find it difficult to balance or to control your pelvis. Engage all the muscles around your pelvis – abdominals, inner thighs, hamstrings, gluteals and pelvic floor – to stabilize. Don't let your pelvis rock back and forth on your sitz bones as you return to the starting position.

· You get the most from this exercise when your movements are controlled, smooth and regular. Work towards this goal by scooping your stomach in and up, squeezing an imaginary ball between your knees and keeping your elbows lifted and wide as you roll. This stabilizes your pelvic and shoulder positions as it curls and strengthens your spine.

Beginner's Modifications for Rolling Like a Ball

As difficult as Rolling Like a Ball can be, it's also an easy exercise to modify; use the modifications in this section of the chapter to make it work for you. With practice, this exercise becomes easier, but it should never be easy. Use these modifications as long as you need to, then drop them to advance. If you have any medical conditions of the spine or pelvis, or other injuries that prevent you from doing this exercise safely, skip this exercise entirely.

Your First Modifications

Keep checking in on your body's ever-changing capabilities as you practise Rolling Like a Ball. Then use any or all of these modifications to help make the exercise challenging, yet accessible, no matter how new to Pilates you might be:

· Eliminate the rolling motion altogether, and focus only on balancing on your tail; use the tips of your toes as props if you need to. Imagine you're inside an inflatable ball, and stretch and conform your body to fill in its inside curve.

· Open up the 'ball' a bit by moving your feet away from your hips and/or moving your hands up your shins. You can even hold the back of your thighs rather than your shins, to open the ball even more (see FIGURE 12-4). When you're ready to add in the rolling movement, you may find that you need to keep this open shape until your spine becomes stronger, more flexible and more uniformly developed. Opening up the ball will help you to focus on scooping your stomach and articulating and massaging your spine.

· If you need a bit of a boost to return to your upright balance after rolling backwards, you can use a slight kicking motion with your lower legs to assist your forward roll. This is a good modification for anyone with uneven tightness in the back, heavier people or pregnant women. Kicking your feet eliminates some of the abdominal strengthening effect of the exercise, but you still get the fantastic spine massage that is one of the key benefits of the Rolling Like a Ball exercise. As your back becomes more flexible, your abdominals will be able to contract better, and you'll be able to stop kicking and make your shape smaller.

· Another approach to modifying is to reduce repetitions.

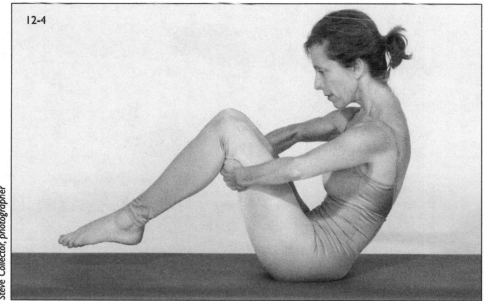

12-4

Steve Collector, photographer

Progressing Beyond the Beginner's Level

As you build skills through practising beginner modifications of Rolling Like a Ball, you can increase the difficulty of the exercise to slowly advance towards the basic intermediate version. Here are some ways to do that:

- If you've started with balancing only, open up the shape and begin rolling.
- Continue this version until you can roll completely to your shoulder blades and return, with no kicks or hand position modifications.
- Gradually decrease the size of your 'ball' by bringing your heels closer to your sitz bones and ears closer to your knees.
- Gradually increase repetitions, up to a maximum of eight.

The Ultimate Version of Rolling Like a Ball

In the ultimate version, your body assumes an even more compact, round shape. Your ears are between your knees, your heels are pulled close to your sitz bones, and your arms firmly hold your body position tighter

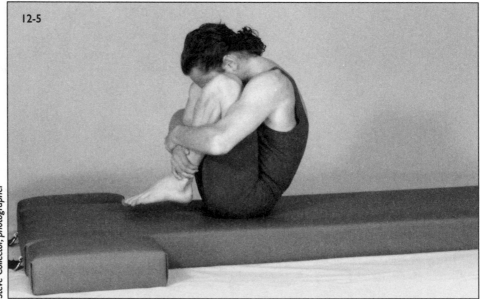

12-5

Steve Collector, photographer

than ever. Pull your legs in powerfully, strengthening and challenging your stomach and shoulder girdle. This action helps further expand and decompress your spine and ribcage as you inhale, and it helps you exhale more deeply to facilitate your forward roll.

To perform the advanced version, grasp your left ankle with your right hand and your right wrist with your left hand (reverse this pattern periodically); maintain this tightly coiled shape as you roll. Keep the elbows high and wide as you squeeze your legs in to you with your arms – this position maintains length in your arm and shoulder girdle muscles as you contract them (see FIGURE 12-5). The oppositional energy of this action balances all the forces around your shoulder girdle and shoulder joints and decompresses your upper spine.

Using Rolling Like a Ball in Other Movements

The Rolling Like a Ball exercise makes you work hard, but it pays off with big benefits. The skills you learn from performing it build coordination and balance, which help you carry out a number of physical tasks simultaneously. If you don't think that's a benefit you'll use too often, consider this: have you ever tried to balance several bags of shopping and a cup of coffee while trying to get the keys out of your pocket so you can unlock your front door? Rolling Like a Ball will make that juggling act a bit easier.

This exercise also increases your spine's flexibility, so you can comfortably and safely reach for objects on high shelves, under your desk, behind your chair or back under the car seat – yes, you can finally retrieve that pen that rolled under there! The strength you build in your hamstrings and gluteal muscles as you practise Rolling Like a Ball will help you with movements as common as walking up the stairs and as challenging as rock climbing or mountain biking. This exercise also builds strength in your shoulder girdle, legs and Powerhouse – a combination you'll use whenever you shovel snow or dig in a garden.

Rolling Like a Ball is a perfect exercise for gymnasts, speed skaters and mountain bikers, all of whom need the balance, coordination, spinal flexibility, abdominal strength and hip and shoulder power that comes from this exercise.

You'll use the skills you learn in Rolling Like a Ball to perform advanced Pilates exercises, such as the Cat on the Trapeze Table or Low Chair, Inversions on the Trapeze Table and Knee Stretches on the Universal Reformer. When you do Knee Stretches, you use oppositional energy to reach your head and coccyx away from each other and to reach your knees towards your head as they pull the Reformer carriage in (see FIGURE 12-6). All the muscles around your pelvis are actively engaged and hold your pelvis suspended above the ground. Your abdominals support the weight and control the shape of your spine as you move your legs, and they squeeze the air from your lungs each time you fold your knees. And all this is done with no mat under your back for support or guidance. Even seasoned Pilates experts find this exercise challenging!

'To breathe correctly you must completely exhale and inhale, always trying very hard to "squeeze" every atom of impure air from your lungs in much the same manner that you would wring every drop of water from a wet cloth... the lungs will automatically completely refill themselves with fresh air. This in turn supplies the blood stream with vitally necessary life-giving oxygen.... Soon the entire body is abundantly charged with fresh oxygen, a fact which makes itself instantly known as the revitalized blood reaches the tips of your fingers and toes.'

Joseph Pilates, *Return to Life Through Contrology*

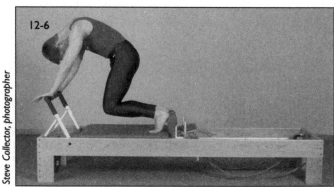

12-6

Steve Collector, photographer

CHAPTER 13

The Single Leg Stretch

Now that you're warmed up – your spine is supple, your abs are firing and you're breathing deeply – you're ready to rock! Both the Single Leg Stretch and the Double Leg Stretch (see Chapter 14) are known as the 'Belly Busters', and with good reason. Both these exercises focus on building the strength and endurance of your abs and your Powerhouse.

What You Need to Know about the Single Leg Stretch

Like the Single Leg Circle, the Single Leg Stretch is an asymmetrical exercise, so it builds upon the skills you developed earlier in that part of your workout. And it incorporates and enhances the resistance training benefit you began developing in the Rolling Like a Ball exercise.

The Single Leg Stretch steps up the heat of your Pilates mat-work session. As you work through this exercise, you'll notice your heart rate increasing and warmth spreading throughout your entire body – there's that internal shower Joseph Pilates felt was so vital! In addition to pumping up your circulation, the Single Leg Stretch introduces new challenges into your workout. The biggest of these is the coordination of all four of your limbs as they move simultaneously and independently of each other. And the exercise encourages you to coordinate your breath and movement in a new, more complicated way. All the new components this exercise brings to your workout help to increase the powerful Pilates benefits you'll gain from the remainder of your session – and the rest of your life!

What Is the Single Leg Stretch?

In the basic Single Leg Stretch, you lie on your back with your upper body and head curled forwards off the mat and one knee bent to your chest, squeezed in with both hands, the other leg stretched out in space on a long diagonal at your working level height. You then switch legs and hand positions, alternately pulling first one knee in to you, then the other as you reach the opposing leg up and away from your torso.

What the Single Leg Stretch Does

Performing the Single Leg Stretch strengthens your Powerhouse and promotes deep Pilates breathing. Here are some additional powerful benefits:

- It elongates your spine while it strengthens and stabilizes your core. Your Powerhouse muscles remain long and strong while they work to stabilize your torso against the opposing energy and force of your limbs reaching out in different directions.

· The simultaneous precise actions of this exercise develop your coordination and mental concentration.

· The asymmetrical actions of your legs and hips build healthy, resilient hip muscles.

· It uniformly develops and centres you by strengthening your core, hips, lower back, shoulders and muscles throughout your entire body.

· It increases your breathing capacity and effectiveness, and thereby improves your circulation.

· It decompresses your spine, hips and shoulders through controlled, flowing movement and oppositional energy as it stimulates your body/mind connection.

The Single Leg Stretch provides a much deeper release and stretch in the hip and lower back than you get from Knee Folds (see Chapters 7 and 8). The Single Leg Stretch movement is much faster, bigger, stronger and more complicated, so it requires more of you, which improves your mastery of Pilates skills and principles.

Tips and Precautions for Doing the Single Leg Stretch

Without question, pelvic stabilization is the most important skill you develop as you do the Single Leg Stretch. All the movements in this exercise challenge you to deepen your understanding and abilities of this important Pilates fundamental skill.

When you do the Single Leg Stretch, your outstretched leg will tend to pull your pelvis into an arch, as your folded leg attempts to draw your pelvis into a tuck and/or move the side of your hip up to your ribs. These destabilizing forces are strongest when you're in the moment of transition, when you let go of one leg and catch the other. Your job is to find a balanced, symmetrical, controllable, safe position for your pelvis and lower back, and to prevent them from either tucking or arching.

Here are some important tips and precautions to keep in mind as you work through the Single Leg Stretch:

· If you hear or feel a clunk or pop as you do the Single Leg Stretch, your body is telling you that you're overworking the front of your thigh and hip muscles or not stabilizing your pelvis effectively. The use of oppositional energy will correct this symptom of overuse, balancing the engagement of all the muscles in order to uniformly develop your muscles and joints.

· If you find that your neck muscles tire quickly, weak abdominal muscles might be causing the problem. When your abs are weak, your neck muscles compensate by taking on an extra load during the Single Leg Stretch. In time your abs will strengthen and this imbalance won't be a problem; until then, try some of the modifications offered later in this chapter.

If you need a refresher on pelvic range of motion and stability, review the relevant sections of Chapters 7 and 8. Also use the imagery and visualization techniques you've learned in other chapters of this book to help master these skills.

· As you curl your upper body forwards in the Single Leg Stretch, draw upon the imagery of the curling wave and the inward-coiling poster to keep your abdominals long. Keep your eyes focused on your scooped stomach. You want to feel elongated – not crunched.

· Use the strength and energy of your whole arm – not just your hands – to pull your bent leg to your torso. The energy of that action engages the muscles throughout your shoulder girdle and reaches into your upper abdominal muscles as well.

· Placing your hands correctly on the shin of your folded leg keeps your knee and hip properly aligned during this exercise. Your hands assume their position quickly during the transition from one leg to the other, so getting the placement right requires coordination and precise control. Practise this part of the exercise on its own, until you can get the placement right without slowing down your transition.

- Your folded leg may angle slightly outwards or inwards when you squeeze it to your body. Experiment to find the position that gives you the best stretch. Does the stretch work better for you if you pull your leg closer to your breastbone or your armpit? Your experimentation might reveal some hidden asymmetries in your hips; consider how these imbalances might be affecting the way you walk, sit or move. Be sure not to tuck.

- You can add a great inner-thigh workout to the Single Leg Stretch through visualization. Imagine that a sheet of glass separates your legs; as you transition from one leg to the other, try to keep both legs in contact with the glass as they pass each other in space. This will engage your entire Powerhouse as well.

- If your knee hurts or you feel an uncomfortable tightness when you squeeze your bent knee in to you with your hands on your shin, try moving your hands to the back of your thigh instead. Don't force your knee to your chest at all costs. As your body becomes more supple, your leg will fold closer to your body. Remember: crushing your body into position doesn't build your skill with this (or any) Pilates exercise.

The Basic Single Leg Stretch Exercise

The steps in the following section outline the basic procedure for performing the Single Leg Stretch at an intermediate level. Prepare to take your time learning this exercise; the coordination of precisely controlled movements can be challenging.

Step by Step Through the Basic Single Leg Stretch

To transition to the Single Leg Stretch, you exhale to return to your upright balancing position, then inhale as you place your left hand on your right shin just below your kneecap (your right hand is still holding your right shin near the ankle). Keep your elbows wide and lifted, and exhale as you roll your spine down to the mat and extend your left leg directly out in line with the centre of your body at your working level height. (Remember the sheet of glass.) Keep your toes softly pointed and your upper body and head curled forwards; focus your eyes on your scooped stomach. (See FIGURE 13-1.)

Now, follow these steps to do the Single Leg Stretch:

1. As you inhale, begin to fold your left knee in and stretch your right leg diagonally out away from you to your working level height; take hold of your left shin and squeeze it to your chest, left hand above the ankle, right hand below the knee, elbows high and wide (see FIGURE 13-2). As you change from one leg to the other, use your concentration and awareness to keep your pelvis and spine stable and maintain your abdominal support. Keep your shoulders open and your elbows high and wide as you squeeze your leg to your chest.

2. Continue inhaling as you switch legs, folding your right knee to your chest and extending your left leg diagonally to your working level height (see FIGURES 13-3 and 13-4). As you bend your leg, imagine that you're playing tug of war with someone who's holding that ankle and

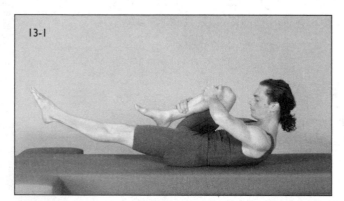

13-3

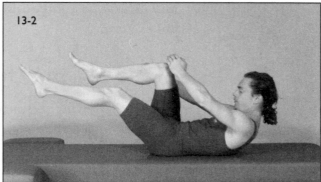

13-2

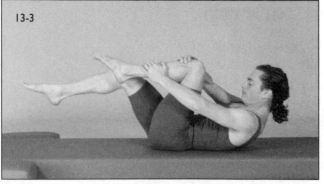

13-1

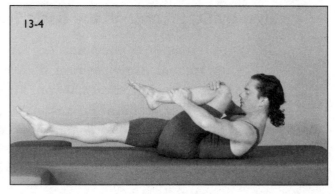

13-4

Steve Collector, photographer

pulling your leg away from you as you bend it. This will stoke the fires of your Powerhouse to build the power to stabilize your spine and pelvis and to strengthen your leg.

3. Exhale as you repeat steps 1 and 2.
4. Repeat steps 1 to 3, four more times, for a total of three inhales and two exhales (ten leg switches), using your final exhale to bend both knees in to your chest. In other words, inhale for two leg switches, then exhale for two leg switches and so on. Don't worry if you do one leg movement more or less!

To get the most from the Single Leg Stretch, use precise, controlled movements and remember to keep your inner legs in contact with that imaginary sheet of glass that separates them. Imagine your extended leg being pulled away from you along a moving walkway; slide the back of your leg along this walkway as it moves away from you to engage your hamstrings and abdominals.

Things to Remember as You Do the Single Leg Stretch

Did the Single Leg Stretch feel like several exercises rolled into one? This exercise calls upon all your Pilates skills, and requires that you closely follow the Pilates guiding principles. Keep these points in mind as you learn this exercise:

· Inhale and exhale completely, wringing your lungs out like a wet sponge. As you squeeze your bent leg to your chest during the exhale phase of the movement, use that pressure to help force the air out of your lungs.
· Engage your body's core muscles deeply and evenly to maintain a stable pelvis and promote uniform development. Your stomach scoop, upper body curl and shoulder/arm engagement form the foundation for that pelvic stability.
· To further stabilize your pelvis, imagine that you're stretching your sitz bones away from your strong Powerhouse; that elongation anchors your pelvis to the mat and keeps it from rocking, arching, tucking or twisting as you switch leg positions.

Smooth, flowing movements improve the efficiency and effectiveness of the Single Leg Stretch. Your goal with this exercise isn't to see how far you can crush your folded leg into your chest. Instead, work towards developing a stable pelvis, increased hip range of motion, long, strong movements and flowing transitions.

Beginner's Modifications for the Single Leg Stretch

The Single Leg Stretch is a challenging exercise, no matter how fit you are or how much experience you have with the Pilates method. If you need some help getting started with the Single Leg Stretch, try some of these modifications. As you gain skill with the exercise, you can work your way towards the basic intermediate version. Then you'll be ready to try some of the advanced modifications to keep the Single Leg Stretch challenging and invigorating.

Your First Modifications

To make the Single Leg Stretch do-able while you're gaining skill with the exercise, try some of these options:

- Reduce repetitions if you become tired.
- If weak abdominals put too much strain on your neck muscles, leave out the upper body curl altogether and lower your spine and head to the mat. When you work with your head lowered, though, you must raise your extended leg straight up into the air – point your toes to the ceiling (see FIGURE 13-5). This position protects your lower back and neck, and enables you to concentrate on practising the leg movements and stabilizing your pelvis without having to hold your head up.
- Use a small pillow to give your head and neck further support. Elevating your head gives you better access to your upper abdominals,

and this will help you to eventually lift your head. However, as you do the Single Leg Stretch with your head on the mat or a pillow, focus on scooping your stomach to build the necessary strength to eventually lift your head. This modified position still gives you a valuable hip stretch as it strengthens your upper abs – and it provides that important Pilates internal shower as you build speed.

Progressing Beyond the Beginner's Level

As your skill with the Single Leg Stretch grows, try using these modifications to advance towards the basic intermediate version of the exercise:

· When you're ready, add the upper body curl into the Single Leg Stretch, but keep your extended leg pointed towards the ceiling.
· Begin lowering your extended leg, but never go lower than your working level. Keep checking your Powerhouse; is your stomach scooped, and are your back and pelvis flat and stable on the mat? Or are they arching and tucking as you switch legs?

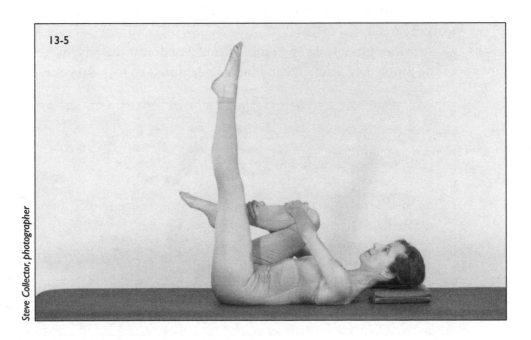

13-5

Steve Collector, photographer

The Ultimate Version of the Single Leg Stretch

When your body is more uniformly developed and you can perform the intermediate version of the Single Leg Stretch without tucking, twisting, rocking or arching your back or pelvis, you're ready for a more advanced movement. Try this:

1. As your bent leg leaves your arms, stretch the tips of your toes to touch the mat, as close to your sitz bones as possible. Slide your toes along the mat until your leg is straight and suspended just a few centimetres above the mat.

2. As you bend the other leg to return it to the bent knee position, slide the tips of those toes back along the mat and pass them as close to your sitz bones as possible (see FIGURE 13-6). The moving walkway and tug-of-war images work well here.

Use your hamstrings to keep your hip joint fully decompressed and mobile during this advanced version of the Single Leg Stretch. As you move through this version, you'll feel those hamstrings heating up and working hard.

Another point to keep in mind: as you're doing the advanced version of the Single Leg Stretch, you might be tempted to lock up your

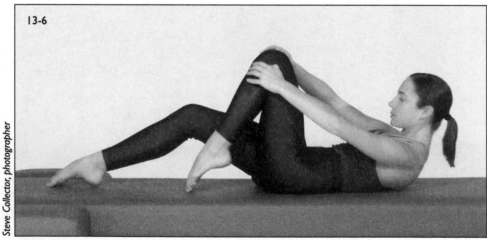

13-6

Steve Collector, photographer

breathing. Keep breathing slowly and completely, and remember not to arch your back or tuck your pelvis. You're giving your whole body – and mind – a workout with this incredible exercise!

Using the Single Leg Stretch in Other Movements

The benefits you gain from doing the Single Leg Stretch extend into every facet of your busy, active life. This exercise develops your body uniformly, so you gain strength, stability and endurance in all of your muscles and joints. The Single Leg Stretch builds a powerful connection between your shoulder girdle and core strength, and you'll feel the power of that benefit when you wash your car, wipe your dinner table, do push-ups or take hold of the handlebars for an extended bicycle ride.

The Single Leg Stretch also increases your hips' range of motion and strengthens your legs, hips and abdomen for deep squatting (remember how you used to squat on the floor as a child, but stopped doing it because getting up became too hard?). In fact, the Single Leg Stretch offers a great way to keep your hips healthy and strong – and healthy hips are essential for remaining active and strong as you age.

This exercise teaches your body to develop strong, precise, coordinated movements as your Powerhouse stabilizes you against the asymmetrical force of your limbs working in opposing directions. You'll use this skill often – when you dance, run, cycle, go rock climbing or practise other sports or exercise programmes that involve jumping, lunging or hurdling. Because the Single Leg Stretch helps you identify and eliminate imbalances in the way you sit, stand and move, it enables you to perform any physical activity with improved strength, grace, balance and control.

You'll take all the benefits of the Single Leg Stretch with you as you move into more advanced Pilates exercises, including the Russian Splits and the Russian Squats on the Universal Reformer and the Up and Down on the Wunda Chair. The skills you developed in the Single Leg Stretch are also essential to performing the Low Chair exercise known as Climb Down the Mountain (see FIGURE 13-8).

In Climb Down the Mountain, you must lift and stabilize your pelvis in space and hold your upper body in a suspended, controlled position as you balance on the ball of one foot. The arms and shoulder girdle actively support your upper body while you vigorously pump the spring-loaded pedal of the chair with the other leg and foot. This exercise requires tremendous strength and flexibility in both hips, along with precise asymmetric control of strong, uniformly developed muscles and joints.

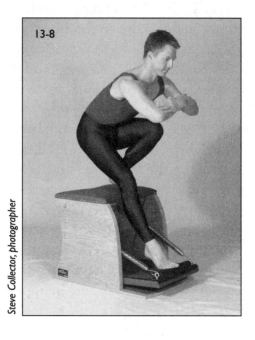

13-8

Steve Collector, photographer

'As we mature, we find ourselves living in bodies not always complementary to our ego. Our bodies are slumped, our shoulders are stooped, our eyes are hollow, our muscles are flabby, and our vitality extremely lowered, if not vanished. This is but the natural result of not having uniformly developed all the muscles of our spine, trunk, arms and legs in the course of pursuing our daily labours and office activities.'

Joseph Pilates, *Return to Life Through Contrology*

CHAPTER 14

The Double Leg Stretch

As you move into your sixth mat-work exercise, you're now in full flow. Take a moment to read your body's messages. Do you have loose or tight hamstrings? Do you overuse the muscles at the front of your thighs? Can you stabilize your pelvis when your legs are moving in space? Is one part of your spine more flexible than another? Are your shoulders and neck feeling stretched – or stressed?

What You Need to Know about the Double Leg Stretch

During the Single Leg Stretch, you challenged your body's ability to remain stable against the force of asymmetrical arm and leg movements. That exercise was an important preparation for the challenges you face at this stage of your Pilates mat-work session. The Double Leg Stretch follows the Single Leg Stretch for a number of reasons. This exercise builds upon and extends the freedom of movement in your hip joints as it requires even more stability in your pelvis and spine than you used in the Single Leg Stretch. And the Double Leg Stretch also builds upon the freedom of movement and stability of your shoulder girdle and arm joints – capabilities you began working on in the Hundred and the Roll-Up.

Unlike the Single Leg Stretch, however, this exercise calls upon your powerful core to support the entire weight of all four of your extended limbs simultaneously. This taxes your stomach beyond anything it has experienced up to this point in your workout. However, if you've been following the Pilates fundamental principles and maintaining your focus on the Pilates goals, you're ready for the challenges.

What Is the Double Leg Stretch?

When you perform the basic Double Leg Stretch, you lie on your back, your upper body and head curled forwards; with a hand on either shin and elbows wide and open, you squeeze both knees to your chest. As in the Single Leg Stretch, you keep your pelvis and lower back long and stable on the mat – no arching or tucking. You then release your shins and simultaneously extend both arms and legs. Your arms reach up and back at a diagonal that extends past your ears, and your legs extend together, out and forwards to your working level height. Then you circle your arms to the side as you bend your legs back into the starting position and take hold of your shins once again.

What the Double Leg Stretch Does

The Double Leg Stretch is a powerful exercise that strengthens your core, legs and upper body, and extends the range of motion of your hip and shoulder joints. This exercise is another perfect example of how Joseph Pilates designed his Contrology movements to facilitate your breathing. Like the motion of an accordion, the extending movements of this exercise help you pull air into your lungs, while the curling and bending motions encourage you to squeeze out as much air as possible.

Tips and Precautions for Doing the Double Leg Stretch

Even the most seasoned Pilates pro must follow a few basic guidelines to get the most from this exercise. Remember these tips and precautions:

· Coil your upper spine into the curl (like a rolled poster or a wave); don't crunch your abs.
· Maintain focus on these three Double Leg Stretch essentials: don't arch your back, scrunch your shoulders or fall back out of your upper body curl.
· Keep your legs at your working height – the height you can suspend your legs above the mat without arching your back or tucking your pelvis. Core stabilization – keeping your entire pelvis and lower spine still and stretched out along the mat – is essential.
· Further aid your core stability by engaging all the muscles around your hips, pelvis and lower back, including your abdominals, gluteals, hamstrings, inner thighs, pelvic floor muscles and the deep hip rotator muscles that connect your sitz bones to your femurs.
· Focus on squeezing your inner thighs tightly together – making your legs 'one' – as you move your legs in the Double Leg Stretch; this action engages the muscles of your pelvic floor, hips and lower abdomen.
· Concentrate on stretching your sitz bones parallel to the mat and away from your scooping stomach and ribcage throughout the entire

Double Leg Stretch; don't let sitz bones point up (pelvic tuck) as you bend your knees, or down (pelvic arch) as you stretch your legs away.

· To achieve a good stretch as you extend your arms and legs in the Double Leg Stretch, imagine that one person has your feet, another has your hands, and the two are pulling you in opposite directions, lengthening your entire body. Gently resist the pulling action by engaging your stomach and pulling your shoulder blades down. Then imagine that the people have released your limbs and you have to maintain the pulling and anchoring energy yourself.

· When you return to your curled position in the Double Leg Stretch, reach your sitz bones parallel to the mat away from your spine and knees. This encourages a deep flexing action that will eliminate bulk in your hip flexors and increase your hips' range of motion.

· Keep your eyes on your scooped stomach at all times. Don't let your head fall backwards as you extend your arms.

The Basic Double Leg Stretch Exercise

The steps in the following section outline the basic procedure for doing the intermediate-level Double Leg Stretch. When you first attempt this exercise, your movements may be awkward and uncertain. That's only natural; over time, as your core strength improves, you'll be better able to flow smoothly through the movements of this exercise.

Step by Step Through the Basic Double Leg Stretch

To transition to the Double Leg Stretch, you exhale to fold your right knee in to your chest to meet your left; place your right hand on your right shin above the ankle; your left hand is still on your left shin above the ankle (see FIGURE 14-1). Now, follow these steps to do the basic intermediate version of the Double Leg Stretch:

1. Inhale to scoop your stomach even deeper as you squeeze your legs together and extend them both in a straight, diagonal line to your working height (toes are softly pointed); at the same time, maintain your upper ab curl as you stretch your arms out and up, in a diagonal

line that runs past your ears (see FIGURES 14-2 and 14-3).

2. Exhale as you circle your arms wide and around to the sides as you bend your knees back in (see FIGURE 14-4); then take hold of both shins and squeeze them together and into your chest to squeeze out every atom of air. Keep your eyes on your stomach, your elbows lifted and wide, and your pelvis stable – don't tuck!

3. Repeat steps 1 and 2 four more times, for a total of five repetitions.

Things to Remember as You Do the Double Leg Stretch

The Double Leg Stretch makes many demands on your Pilates skills. You have to maintain stability, core strength and flowing movement while extending and contracting all of your limbs. To make the most progress (and get the most benefit), keep these points in mind:

· Maintain your upper body curl as you extend your arms away from your body – don't let your upper body fall back in space.

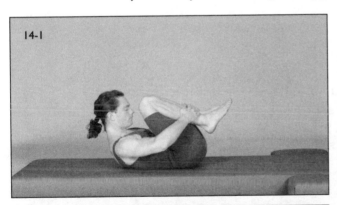

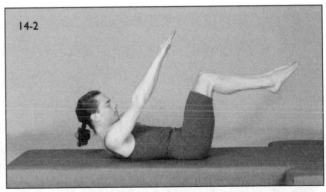

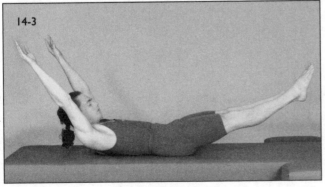

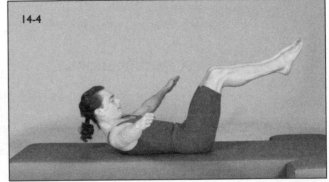

Steve Collector, photographer

- If you have weak abdominals and lower-back muscles or tight hip flexors, you may have trouble maintaining good core stability. In the beginning, be certain to keep your legs high enough to be able to stabilize your spine and pelvis.
- Keep your arms in your peripheral vision as you bring them back around to grasp your bent legs. In other words, you should be able to see your arms moving towards your sides without turning your head. This practice promotes healthy neck and shoulder placement, and prevents shoulder muscle strain.
- Keep your shoulders down as you reach your arms away from your body, and keep your elbows lifted and wide as you squeeze your knees to your chest.
- To avoid overusing the muscles at the front of your hips, use the image of the moving walkway or ramp that you learned in Chapter 13. That visualization will help you engage your hamstrings and stomach, and reduce your reliance on your hip flexors.

Beginner's Modifications for the Double Leg Stretch

Having trouble with the basic intermediate version of the Double Leg Stretch? Don't be disappointed; many people do when they first learn this exercise. Your goal is to develop full-body strength and a deeper level of core power as you increase the strength and range of motion in your hips and shoulders. With these goals in mind, you can use any of the modifications listed in this section to help you begin mastering the Double Leg Stretch. In time you'll advance through the intermediate version, and then it's on to the advanced challenge!

Your First Modifications

Here are some beginner-level modifications that keep the Double Leg Stretch challenging while making it a bit more approachable:

- Reduce repetitions or rest in between repetitions if your neck or stomach get tired.
- To reduce neck fatigue, eliminate the upper ab curl and lower your head to the mat (use a small pillow if you need additional support). If you lower your head, however, you must raise your legs to a 90-degree angle from the mat to prevent strain on your neck or lower back. Stretch your legs and arms straight up in the air, fingers and toes pointing to the ceiling (see FIGURE 14-5). This modification works well as you build strength in your abdominals and lower-back muscles.
- In this position, practise the leg and arm movements as you focus on maintaining the spine and pelvic stability necessary for the exercise. Scoop your stomach deeper with each repetition to help with this stabilization and maintain a brisk pace. Even in this modified position, the exercise gives you a valuable hip stretch, upper abdominal strengthening and the ever-important internal shower.
- Do only the upper body curl and arm circles while resting your feet on the mat, knees bent and legs together. This modification draws upon

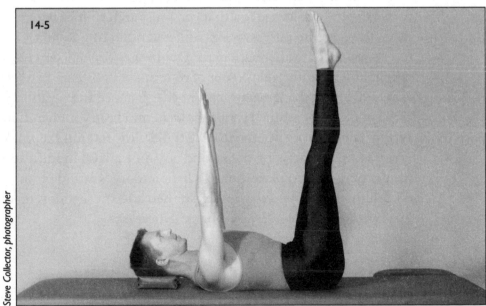

14-5

Steve Collector, photographer

the fundamental movements of the ribcage arms and upper body curls (see Chapters 7 and 8 to review the details).

Progressing Beyond the Beginner's Level

As your skills and strength build, you can use any of these modifications to work towards mastering the intermediate version of the Double Leg Stretch exercise:

· If you've been working with your head lowered to the mat or resting on a pillow, add the upper ab curl, but keep your legs and arms extended up towards the ceiling.

· Next, add leg movements; begin by extending your legs towards the ceiling; as you develop increased core strength, try lowering the angle of your legs. Eventually, you should be able to work with your legs at a 45-degree angle to the mat.

· As you work to lower your legs, begin gradually reaching backwards with your arms until they can comfortably stretch backwards diagonally at an angle that runs past your ears (you developed this same skill when you worked through the Roll-Up in Chapter 10). Never try to force yourself to work with your legs so low that you must arch your back or tilt your pelvis. It's better to raise your legs a bit and build core strength.

As you reach farther back in the Double Leg Stretch, don't let the weight of your arms pull you out of your upper body curl. Extend your arms and legs at the same height for better balance and position. Don't arch your back or scrunch your shoulders, and keep your hands in your peripheral vision, no matter how big the circling motion they make.

· If you've been practising the second beginning-level modification (upper body curl in place, but legs bent and feet resting on the mat), try folding your knees to your chest; then add the leg movement (beginning at 90 degrees) as your skill increases.

The Ultimate Version
of the Double Leg Stretch

As you continue to practise the Double Leg Stretch, you will build strength and skill; eventually you'll be ready to move beyond the intermediate version. When you want to take the Double Leg Stretch even further, try these modifications:

· In time your abdominals become more powerful and supple, so you can extend your legs at a lower angle. Try to build towards a working level height of 7.5cm (3in) above the mat, or eye height.

· Extend the range of motion of your arms until they move behind your ears and head; remember not to lean back or lift your ribs or shoulders as you circle your arms.

· Finally, add the toe slide you learned in Chapter 13. When you begin your leg extension, reach with the tips of your toes for the mat. Touch the mat as close to your sitz bones as possible, then slide your toes away from you along the mat until your legs are straight and just 7.5cm (3in) above the mat (see FIGURE 14-6). Keep elongating your entire body as if you're being pulled apart, even as you return your legs to their bent position; slide your toes back along the mat until they are as close to your sitz bones as possible, then bend your legs into your encircling arms. The moving walkway image works well here, too.

As you add these modifications, you can congratulate yourself on how incredibly flexible and powerful you have become!

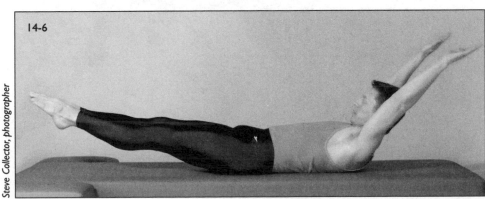

14-6

Steve Collector, photographer

Using the Double Leg Stretch in Other Movements

The Double Leg Stretch delivers the same sort of fitness benefits you get from the Single Leg Stretch, but in double doses! This exercise increases the strength and range of motion in your shoulder girdle, so you can reach higher, lift more efficiently and maintain better strength and balance in every extended movement you make. The Double Leg Stretch is also a terrific way to build strength and flexibility in your hips. You'll feel those benefits every time you stoop to pick up a child, get out of the bath, push a heavy mower up a hill or squat to sit on the floor (and then get up again).

This exercise is a great aid in developing deep, healthy breathing, a skill necessary for a healthy life and of particular interest to high-altitude athletes such as hikers and skiers. And any athlete (weekend or otherwise) will benefit from the increased strength, stability and endurance this exercise promotes, whether you're cycling through the countryside, smashing a tennis ball, swimming, playing catch or reaching for holds during rock climbing.

The skills you develop in the Double Leg Stretch are integral to many advanced Pilates movements, including the Flying Arm Springs on the Trapeze Table (shown in FIGURE 14-7), Control Push-Ups on the Universal Reformer and the Handstand Pike on the Low Chair, to name just a few.

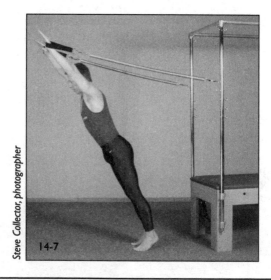

Steve Collector, photographer

14-7

CHAPTER 15

The Spine Stretch

At this point in your Pilates workout, you've just finished two intense gut-busting exercises – the Single and Double Leg Stretches. Now, your body's ready for a change of both pace and space. You've been lying down and working to stabilize your spine and pelvis, and now you get to sit up in the waterfall of gravity, and align and stretch your spine in a new, powerful orientation.

What You Need to Know about the Spine Stretch

Although all Pilates exercises promote both stability and flexibility through simultaneously strengthening, stretching and uniformly developing your musculature, each exercise has a primary focus. The order of these exercises throughout the mat-work series alternates the focus – on either strengthening, stretching, stabilizing or articulating. The Hundred focuses primarily on building strength and stability in your Powerhouse; the Roll-Up stretches and articulates your spine; the Single Leg Circle builds strength and stability in your spine by requiring it to counter the asymmetrical effect of your leg circling in space; Rolling Like A Ball once again massages and stretches the muscles of your back; the Single and Double Leg Stretches strengthen your spine and abdominals by requiring them to work hard to stabilize against the moving weight of your extended legs.

The Spine Stretch elongates and decompresses your spine and helps you to breathe deeply and fully. These benefits make the Spine Stretch a perfect exercise for anyone who sits in front of a computer all day. Use a few repetitions of this exercise to revitalize your body during your working day (do it sitting in your chair if you can't get on the floor at work).

The Spine Stretch fits nicely into this pattern by returning emphasis to stretching and articulating your joints and muscles to release any tension and tightness you might have developed during your workout. During the Spine Stretch, your spine is upright and supported by your Powerhouse instead of a mat, so it can enjoy a new freedom of movement. Your legs and hips are supported on the floor, so your hips can flex freely and enable you to sit upright on top of your sitz bones in good pelvic alignment without tightness or tension. The Spine Stretch offers your body an opportunity to regroup its strength and find refreshment in a calm, yet powerful, exercise.

What Is the Spine Stretch?

In the basic intermediate Spine Stretch exercise, you sit upright on the mat with your legs extended before you in a V-shape (the official Pilates mat includes foot boxes designed to guide your legs into the correct position). You extend your arms out in front of you, at shoulder height and width, then exhale as you stretch by curling your spine forwards and over towards the mat. As you return to an upright position, your lungs automatically completely refill themselves with fresh air.

What the Spine Stretch Does

As you've read, the Spine Stretch focuses primarily on stretching your spine's muscles and joints to make them more flexible. But this exercise, like all Pilates movements, has a number of other benefits, as well:

· It encourages you to use your Powerhouse to promote deep Pilates breathing.
· It stretches your hamstrings, gluteals and lower back. As mentioned earlier, tight hamstrings restrict your hip and spine movements and can lead to ineffective movement patterns and overuse injuries.
· It strengthens and balances all the muscles in your Powerhouse and pelvis, including your abdominals, hips, lower back, pelvic floor, deep hip rotators and inner thighs, as well as your hamstrings.
· It improves your posture by aligning your vertebrae in the waterfall of gravity and increasing your spine's strength, length and flexibility.
· It increases shoulder stability and range of motion, as well as pelvic stability and control.
· It teaches you to separate and individually control the movements of your arms, ribs, shoulders and neck – important for preventing neck, shoulder and arm injury.
· It calms and focuses your body, mind and spirit; the simplicity of the exercise allows you to control and balance the activity level of your mind.

Tips and Precautions for Doing the Spine Stretch

The Spine Stretch is calming and comforting, but it's still a powerful exercise. Follow these tips and precautions to get the most from it:

- If you can't sit upright on top of your sitz bones easily because your hamstrings and/or hip flexors are too tight, sit on a low box, phone book or rolled-up towel, or bend your knees slightly, until the necessary muscles lengthen.
- Keep your shoulders down and wide; don't allow them to lift or round forwards into your chest as you curl your spine.
- Concentrate on articulating your spine one vertebra at a time. As you stretch forwards, don't just lean over. Use the wave image to lengthen, lift and decompress your spine during this movement, so you don't crunch and shorten your abs. As you uncurl, use your abdominal muscles and the power of your inhalation to lift and stack each vertebra onto the preceding one, rather than pulling your spine up with your back muscles.
- Keep your knees facing straight up – don't let your legs roll in or out. This will help you stretch tight leg, hip and lower-back muscles, and enable you to better strengthen your lower abdominals, *iliopsoas* and pelvic floor muscles.
- Exhale fully and steadily with an open mouth so you don't grip or catch your breath. Be sure to squeeze all the air out of your lungs.
- Keep elbows and knees extended but relaxed – don't lock them. Keep your heels on the mat.
- Imagine your spine is rising like a tall tree, so your lifting-up movement is powerful and controlled. Allow the front of your ribs to be softly knitted together. Don't arch or tighten your mid-back by thrusting the ribs forwards to hold yourself up. Feel gravity's waterfall coursing through your aligned bones.

Prop a mirror up beside you and watch as you do the Spine Stretch. Look for inefficient movement habits and for spots where your spine doesn't bend or bends too much (you may be bending too much at your neck, upper back or hip). Use this information to correct your movement patterns and to loosen up those rigid spots in your spine.

The Basic Spine Stretch Exercise

The Spine Stretch calls upon your skills in the fundamental movements you learned in Chapters 7 and 8. If you need refreshing on these skills, reread these chapters before you begin the Spine Stretch.

Step by Step Through the Basic Spine Stretch

Complete your last Double Leg Stretch by exhaling, then inhale as you move your right hand onto your left shin and slide your right leg out along the mat. Press your left shin into both hands and exhale as you roll up to a sitting position. Inhale as you extend both legs out in front of you in a V-shape, with your feet about 1m (3ft) apart; keep your knees facing up towards the ceiling and your ankles softly flexed. Exhale as you raise your straight arms in front of you, parallel to the ground, shoulder height and width, palms down (see FIGURE 15-1).

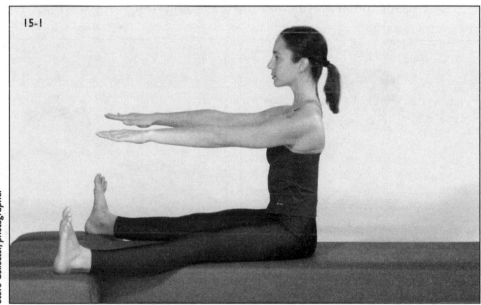

15-1

Steve Collector, photographer

Now follow these steps to perform the basic intermediate Spine Stretch:

1. Inhale to scoop your stomach in and up along the front of your spine; fill your lungs completely to expand your ribs and decompress your spine (keep the opening umbrella image in mind).

2. Exhale as you curl first your head, and then your spine up and over towards the mat, like a wave cresting over a surfer, with each vertebra individually following your head in a flowing forward movement (see FIGURE 15-2). Continue curling your upper body forwards until your entire spine is rounded and the top of your head is as close to the mat as possible (see FIGURE 15-3). Keep your knees straight and use your curling movement to wring all of the air from your lungs.

3. Begin to inhale as you press your hamstrings down into the mat (without tucking) and, starting at your pubic bone, pull your stomach in and up to stack one vertebra upon the next sequentially, returning to your upright position. Imagine that you're lightly pressing each vertebra up along a wall behind you as you rise. When you're fully erect, your lungs will be completely inflated, your ribs expanded in all directions, and your spine elongated and decompressed.

4. Repeat steps 2 and 3 four more times, increasing your stretch, refining your spinal articulation and deepening your scoop with each repetition.

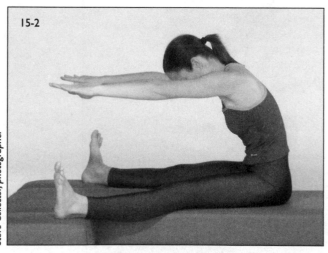

15-2

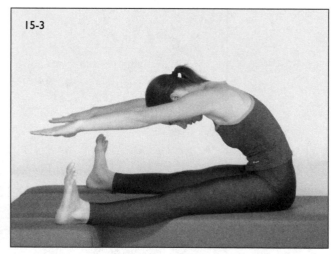

15-3

Steve Collector, photographer

Things to Remember as You Do the Spine Stretch

You get the most from the Spine Stretch when you remember and follow the guiding principles of Pilates during each movement of the exercise:

· While you concentrate on the specific details of each movement within the exercise, be aware of your body as a whole.

· Use your scooped stomach to help centre your energy.

· Focus on the precise control of your forward movement to curl and uncurl your spine one vertebra at a time, and use this control to keep all your movements flowing and natural.

· Feel the oppositional energy between your upper body's forward motion and your firmly anchored legs and feet. Remember to press your hamstrings down into and along the mat without tucking as your Powerhouse lifts, curls and uncurls, and notice the stretch as your arms and legs pull in opposite directions from your body's centre.

· And finally, remember to use your breathing to help curl and uncurl your upper body, and to expand and separate your ribs and vertebrae. Notice where you put your breath and how the breath helps you move and how the movement helps you breathe. Time your exhalation so that your curl squeezes the last bit of air out of your lungs, and time your inhalation so that your lungs are at full capacity as your spine finishes its upward movement.

Beginner's Modifications for the Spine Stretch

Your range of motion, spinal flexibility and breathing capacity will grow with each repetition of the Spine Stretch, but in the beginning you may have problems performing the intermediate version. As you already know, you can modify any of the exercises in this book with three basic changes: reducing the number of repetitions, the range of motion or the load required of specific muscles or joints.

Use the modifications presented in this section of the chapter to make the Spine Stretch more do-able, while still working towards the goals of increasing your spine's flexibility, building strong, long hamstrings and developing your Powerhouse to promote deep, healthy Pilates breathing:

- If you feel tension or strain in your neck or shoulders, place your palms on the mat between your thighs and allow them to slide forwards and backwards along the mat as your curl and uncurl.

- If you feel pain or uncomfortable pulling in your hips, lower back, knees or thighs when you sit upright with your legs straight out before you, your hips or hamstrings probably are too tight. The Spine Stretch works to solve that problem, but until your body grows more supple, you can alleviate the discomfort by elevating your hips. Do so by sitting on a low box, phone book, small pillow or folded towel (see FIGURE 15-4). If your hamstrings are very tight, try sitting on a chair or stairway as you do the Spine Stretch. Relax your ankles into a soft point.

- You also can bend your knees slightly to alleviate some of the pull on the hamstrings and lower back. Don't bend your knees so much that

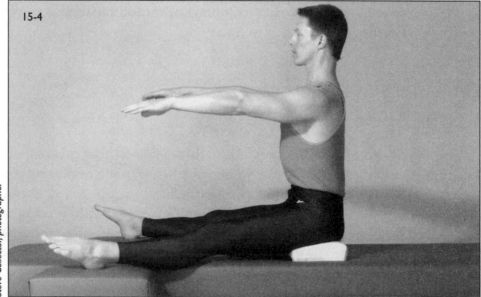

15-4

Steve Collector, photographer

your pelvis tucks under more; bend them just enough to enable your pelvis to sit upright.

· Curl forwards only as far as is comfortable for you; your range of motion will increase as you become more flexible.

The Ultimate Version of the Spine Stretch

As your body becomes more uniformly developed, you can continue to keep this exercise challenging in several ways:

· Flex your ankles and toes powerfully back towards your knees to increase the stretch on your calves, hamstrings and back. Keep your knees pointed towards the ceiling and your heels on the mat.

· Begin the Spine Stretch with your arms extended above your head beside your ears (see FIGURE 15-5). This position strengthens your shoulder girdle and increases its stretch; in addition, it allows you to breathe deeply and fully. This position will challenge and strengthen your abdominals to keep your spine and ribcage from arching as you lift your arms.

· Curl your spine even deeper, as if you're trying to put the back of your head on the mat as close to you as possible (see FIGURE 15-6). Increasing the curl in your spine will make your spine feel young, no matter how old you are.

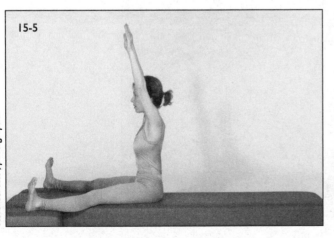

15-5

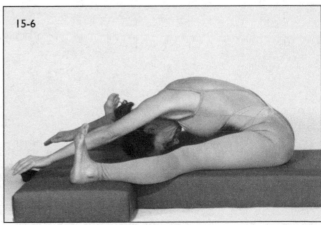

15-6

Steve Collector, photographer

Using the Spine Stretch
in Other Movements

The Spine Stretch is all about building a healthier, stronger and more flexible spine. Joseph Pilates designed many exercises, including the Roll-Up and Rolling Like a Ball, to promote this fitness goal. As he said in *Return to Life Through Contrology*, a healthy spine's 'flexibility would be comparable to that of the finest watch spring steel'. A healthy, flexible spine enables you to engage your abdominal muscles, supports your organs and gives them more 'working' room, and helps you breathe more deeply.

Everyone – from the most highly trained athlete to the home gardener or computer programmer – benefits from these fitness improvements. A mother who frequently has to bend down to pick up her 14kg (30lb) three-year-old needs a 'watch spring' spine, a healthy, 'smart' shoulder girdle and strong, long hamstrings, and so does an Olympic hurdler. Imagine that hurdler, for a moment, as she leaps forward, front leg reaching long and high, spine lifting and curling forwards to propel her body over the hurdle and prepare for a balanced landing; with the skills

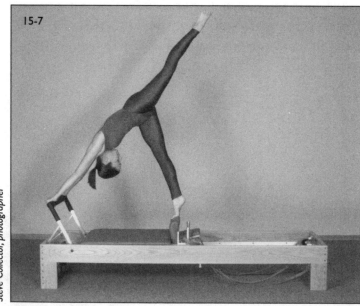

15-7

Steve Collector, photographer

developed in regular practice with the Spine Stretch, that hurdler lands safely and efficiently, never losing stride or speed.

With regular practice of the Spine Stretch, you'll find yourself moving closer every day to the central Pilates goal of a uniformly developed body, mind and spirit. And this exercise also helps your progress towards more advanced Pilates movements and exercises, such as the Open Leg Rocker on the Mat; the Push Through Series on the Trapeze Table; the Jackknife and Pike on the Low Chair, and the Elephant and Arabesque on the Universal Reformer. (FIGURE 15-7 illustrates the Arabesque on the Shoulder Blocks on the Universal Reformer, an exciting advanced Pilates exercise you work towards with the Spine Stretch).

'As a heavy rainstorm freshens the water of a sluggish or stagnant stream and whips it into immediate action, so Contrology exercises purify the blood in the bloodstream and whip it into instant action with the result that the organs of the body... receive the benefit of clean fresh blood carried to them by the rejuvenated bloodstream.'

Joseph Pilates, *Return to Life Through Contrology*

CHAPTER 16

The Saw

The Saw is the first intermediate-level mat-work exercise that twists the spine. It requires you to coordinate movements in your shoulders, pelvis, hips and spine. This total-body workout feels great and will move you further towards the Pilates goal of uniform development – so enjoy as you learn!

What You Need to Know about the Saw

As you work through the complete series of Pilates mat-work exercises, you will discover that each exercise builds upon those that precede it. In other words, the skills you learn in each exercise develop your body/mind fitness, advancing your capabilities towards the next exercise – and the next fitness level.

The Hundred and the Roll-Up exercises you learned in Chapters 9 and 10 prepare you for the Saw by stabilizing your pelvis, strengthening your abdominals, and stretching and massaging your upper back (both to warm up its muscles and to promote deep Pilates breathing). The Single Leg Circle you learned in Chapter 11 elongates your torso, teaches you to integrate and coordinate your movements, and improves your ability to stabilize your body during asymmetrical movements (and even incorporates a small twisting motion of the lower spine and pelvis in its advanced version). The Rolling Like a Ball exercise (Chapter 12) further develops your spine's flexibility. The Single and Double Leg Stretches (Chapters 13 and 14) continue developing your abilities to stabilize your body during asymmetrical movements as they stretch your spine and increase the fullness of your breathing.

The stretching and twisting motion of the Saw wrings the air out of your lungs, then helps inflate and refill them. This wringing and automatic refilling action is very like what you experienced in the Spine Stretch (see Chapter 15).

The Spine Stretch is the perfect precursor to the Saw. The Spine Stretch increases your spine's length, strength and flexibility as it stretches your ribs open and decompresses your vertebrae to give your lungs and organs lots of room to do their jobs. You take all of these skills even further in the Saw, as you twist and flex your torso. This twisting motion improves your breathing as it challenges you anew and increases the flexibility of your spine, hips and shoulders.

What Is the Saw?

The Saw involves twisting to reach the fingers of one hand towards the toes of the opposite foot. You perform the Saw in a sitting position, legs extended before you in a V, arms extended straight out to either side at shoulder height, with palms facing down. Timing your inhalations and exhalations with your movements, you first twist your torso then curl forwards, reaching your hand for the opposite foot; the other hand raises up behind you. The Saw twists and bends towards alternate sides to provide uniform development and maximum flexibility.

What the Saw Does

The twisting motion of the Saw is powerful in a number of ways. It stretches your back, hips and shoulders, increasing your range of motion and improving your breath capacity. It also stimulates your nervous system by rotating and elongating your spine (the structure that houses your spinal cord). This intricate movement involves many joints, including your shoulder and shoulder girdle, pelvis, hips and all your vertebrae. Because this twisting motion has such wide-ranging impact, it requires that you very skilfully control your movements and pay close attention to the stability and flexibility of your pelvis, spine and shoulders.

Of course, the primary goal of the Saw – as in so many Pilates exercises – is to expand your lungs and chest so you can breathe more fully. The Saw's twisting motion wrings stale, used air out of your lungs, just as you wring water from a dishcloth. In addition to these primary goals, the Saw provides several other valuable benefits:

· The Saw's twisting action helps flush toxins from your blood by encouraging robust breathing and circulation.
· It strengthens the muscles in your abdominal corset, especially the internal and external obliques.
· It promotes the development of greater pelvic and shoulder girdle stability by training your body through complicated mechanical motions.

- It increases the range of motion in your spine and shoulders by stretching and twisting the muscles surrounding them further and in a new way.
- It uses the movements of your arm and shoulder girdle to help increase the strength and flexibility of your back and Powerhouse.
- Because of its asymmetric nature, the Saw helps improve your body's uniform development by revealing muscle/joint imbalances or inflexibilities not exposed by earlier exercises in this series.
- It stretches the muscles along the sides of your torso, to prepare you for later exercises, such as the Swan and the Side Kicks.

Tips and Precautions for Doing the Saw

As you prepare to do the Saw, keep these points in mind:

- You should be able to sit upright on your sitz bones comfortably; if you cannot, use one of the beginner-level modifications offered later in the chapter.
- To engage your obliques most effectively, scoop your stomach in and up along the front of your spine and begin the twist at your coccyx rather than your shoulder girdle. Keep your pelvis stable.
- Allow your front arm to move across your body only as far as needed to reach for your opposite foot; get most of your reaching range from your spine, rather than your arms.
- As you move the arm to the back, first sweep it downwards past your hip before lifting it up behind you; this approach helps to protect the shoulder from strain.
- Keep the forward hand level with your toes to strengthen your shoulder girdle and abs more effectively – don't let it drop to the floor.
- Each time you return to your upright position (between each reach), stack your spine straight up. Avoid leaning backwards or forwards – imagine that you're stacking each vertebra on the one below it, and as you add each vertebra to the stack, you're lightly pressing it up along a wall behind you.
- To activate your Powerhouse, press your hamstrings down into the mat, without tucking, and then away from your sitz bones towards your feet.

- · Throughout the entire exercise, stretch the fingertips of each hand away from those of the other; this action engages your Powerhouse muscles and stretches and strengthens your shoulder girdle.
- · Keep both sitz bones firmly planted on the mat at all times so that you twist your spine and not your pelvis.

The Basic Saw Exercise

The steps in the section that follows offer the basic intermediate version of the Saw. If you need beginner-level modifications, you'll find those in the next section. If you're sufficiently uniformly developed to require a more challenging routine, refer to the advanced modifications further on in the chapter.

Step by Step Through the Basic Saw

Finish the Spine Stretch, and exhale as you open your arms to your sides, reaching straight out with them as if you're trying to touch opposite walls. Keep them in your peripheral vision, at shoulder height, with palms facing down and elbows soft and unlocked (see FIGURE 16-1).

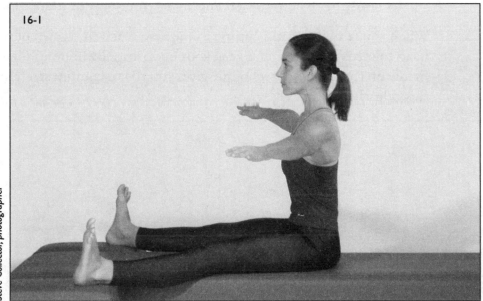

16-1

Steve Collector, photographer

Now follow these steps:

1. Inhale as you press your hamstrings down into the mat and lift your abdominals in and up to lengthen your spine as you twist your spine and upper body to the left (see FIGURE 16-2). Keep your right hip and sitz bone anchored to the mat as you begin the twist from your tailbone and feel it spiral up through each vertebra to the crown of your head.

2. Exhale as you arc the crown of your head, and then spine, vertebra by vertebra, over your left leg, like a wave curling up and over a surfer. Rotate your left arm inward, sweeping it first down towards the floor, then up behind you, palm facing up to the ceiling, as your right hand reaches towards your left foot (see FIGURE 16-3). Allow the fingers of your right hand to 'saw' against your left little toe at the furthest point of this stretch.

3. Inhale, pressing your hamstrings down into the mat to engage your deepest pelvic and abdominal muscles, and begin lifting and turning your spine and Powerhouse back through centre and continuing to the right. Fully inflate your lungs with fresh, clean air as you stack each vertebra on top of the one below it, building your posture and your Powerhouse back up to a centred, upright position.

4. Repeat steps 2 and 3, working to the right side, then repeat the entire set (twisting to both the left and right) three or four more times.

When you're twisting and curling in the Saw, reach the crown of your head towards your shin, and keep your opposing sitz bone and hamstring firmly on the mat. This technique gives you the maximum stretch and flexibility benefit.

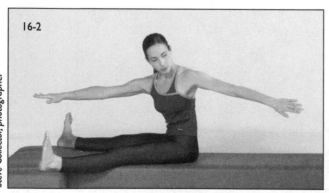

16-2

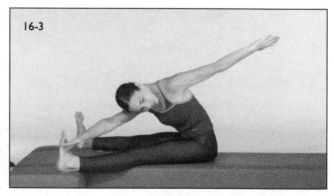

16-3

Things to Remember as You Do the Saw

You'll get more from the Saw if you hold these thoughts as you work through it:

·   Keep your sitz bones anchored and maintain your pelvic stability. Doing so will teach you how to separate the movement of your spine from those of your hips and legs, and will give you a longer, more effective stretch.

·   As you lift the palm held behind you towards the ceiling, you're integrating the movement of your shoulder girdle into an upper body curl (see Chapters 7 and 8) to increase your spine's flexibility.

·   Reach towards your shin with the crown of your head – not your nose or chin – as you twist and curl forwards. Keeping good neck alignment will help you achieve more uniform flexibility and core power.

·   Use the guiding principle of oppositional energy to lift your spine up through the crown of your head and away from your anchored sitz bones. Maintain this feeling throughout the exercise to decompress your spine, engage your Powerhouse and give you more room to breathe.

Beginner's Modifications for the Saw

If you feel uncomfortable as you twist to the side and curl forwards in the Saw, stop and determine where the discomfort or tightness seems to originate. Then use any of the following modification techniques to make the Saw work for you in your current physical condition. However, you should not eliminate the twisting action altogether – it's essential for this exercise.

You can modify the Saw in several ways, including the traditional methods of cutting repetitions or limiting the range of the movements involved in the exercise. As long as you continue to twist your spine, you're still gaining the essential benefit of this exercise. Try these modifications to make the Saw comfortable, while still challenging:

- If your hips or hamstrings are tight, you might have problems sitting comfortably with your legs and feet stretched straight out from your erect torso. In that case, elevate your hips slightly by sitting on a low box, phone book, a Small Barrel or a folded towel (see FIGURE 16-4).
- If you need more elevation, try sitting in a chair or on a stair step; your goal is to be comfortable in an upright position on top of your sitz bones.
- You can alleviate some of the pull on the hamstrings and lower back by bending your knees a bit, but only as much as necessary to enable your pelvis to sit upright (don't tuck). Softly point your toes.
- If the forward curl is too uncomfortable for you at this point, focus on the twisting motion only or limit the forward range of the curl.
- If neck and shoulder tightness is a problem, lower the height of your arms and hands, and limit the forward range of your curl.

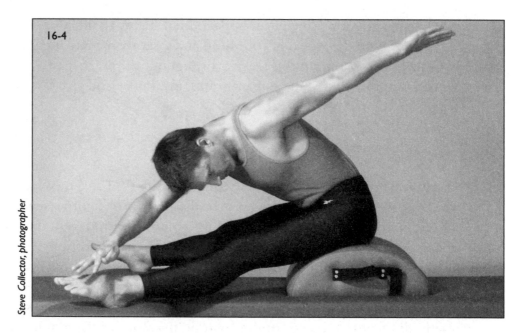

16-4

Steve Collector, photographer

The Ultimate Version of the Saw

As you gain practice with the Saw, your body will become stronger and more uniformly developed. Your spine and hamstrings will grow more flexible, so you can curl more effectively and with better articulation in your spine. Your shoulders and shoulder girdle will become more integrated, stable and flexible, so you can reach further. Your spine will decompress and elongate, allowing you to twist further and breathe more deeply.

When you reach this point, you're ready to take the Saw to more advanced levels. Try these modifications:

- Powerfully flex your feet back towards your body to increase the stretch on your calves, hamstrings and back. When you flex your feet backwards, don't simply shorten the front of your thigh or shin. Imagine that your hamstrings and calves are lengthening so far down along the mat that they push your heels away until your foot curls back into a flex at the ankle. Make sure to keep your knees pointed towards the ceiling and your heels firmly on the mat as you do this flex.
- Curl your spine even deeper, imagining that you're trying to put the back of your head on your upper shin.
- Reach your arms farther apart from one another – the front hand reaching past your little toe and the back palm lifting higher to bend your spine.

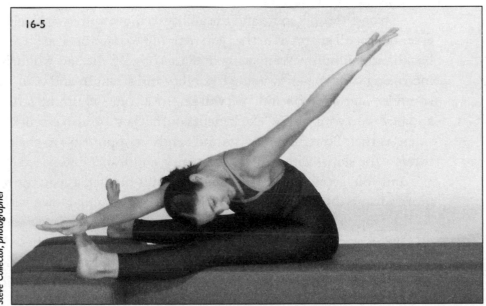

16-5

Steve Collector, photographer

- As you curl, continue twisting your spine until you're looking under your shoulder and towards your back hand (see FIGURE 16-5).
- Finally, at the end of your curl and stretch, add a second squeeze to exhale more air from your lungs and to pulse you further forwards; this small sliding action gives this exercise its name – the Saw!

It's important to realize that increasing the number of repetitions for the Saw is *not* a healthy modification. Five full repetitions (with a curl and stretch to both sides) are enough. Remember that Joseph Pilates designed his exercises very carefully and specifically. You can use fewer than five repetitions if necessary, but don't use more. You can tire your muscles, making your body vulnerable to overuse injuries.

Using the Saw in Other Movements

Most of the activities of daily life involve twisting, turning and bending the spine. You use the benefits gained from practising the Saw every time you get out of bed, move plates in and out of the dishwasher or reach into the back seat of your car. And each season brings new demands for these skills, as you cut firewood, shovel snow, dig up your garden, go swimming and rake the autumn leaves.

A strong, flexible spine and the ability to move and twist freely are essential for all sports. Whether you're trying to develop a stronger backhand or improve your swing in tennis or golf, the Saw will help. By increasing your spine's twisting flexibility and strength and your shoulder's range of motion, you will improve your swimming stroke or add power to your throw. The benefits of the Saw are also essential to skiers as their Powerhouse twists and bends in opposition to their legs to traverse the slopes with control, efficiency, endurance and speed.

And you'll continue to develop these skills further, as you move to more advanced Pilates exercises, including the Hanging Down with Twist on the Trapeze Table; the Twist on the Reformer; Sitting Twist and Twist on Hip on the Low Chair; and Twist I and II on the mat. All these exercises require the twisting, flexing, stabilizing and strengthening skills you develop with regular practice of the Saw as part of your complete

Pilates mat-work programme. (FIGURE 16-6 illustrates Twist I on the mat, an exercise that requires you to perform the Saw's crucial skills balanced on one hand and one foot!)

> 'By reawakening thousands and thousands of ordinarily dormant muscle cells, Contrology correspondingly reawakens thousands and thousands of dormant brain cells, thus activating new areas and stimulating further the functioning of the mind. No wonder then that so many persons express such great surprise following their initial experience.... For the first time in many years their minds have been truly awakened.'

> Joseph Pilates, *Return to Life Through Contrology*

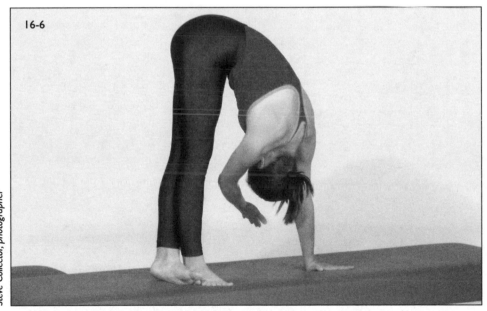

16-6

Steve Collector, photographer

CHAPTER 17

The Swan

The next exercise in the Pilates mat-work series, the Swan, introduces a new spine-extending, backward-bending movement to help develop skills and muscles that are unworked (or under-worked) in your daily life. By building your ability to extend your torso backwards, you're moving closer to the important Pilates goal of uniform development. And the Swan feels good, too!

What You Need to Know about the Swan

Throughout this book, you've read of the importance of keeping your body erect and well aligned. When your body is well-balanced and properly aligned, you stand and move in concert with the force of gravity, rather than resisting it. A long, strong, flexible spine makes all your movements more graceful, balanced and efficient. You breathe more deeply and feel more active and alert.

When you're stooped and bent, you encourage your muscles and joints to tighten up and grow stiff with disuse. Your posture is slouched, your abdomen falls forwards and your hips and shoulders ache. Your hip flexors and inner thighs tighten and shorten, pulling your pelvis out of alignment and stressing your back even further.

Joseph Pilates bemoaned the 'thousands of persons with round, stooped shoulders and protruding abdomens' he saw around him, because he knew this condition would eliminate any hope for these people to lead full, active, healthy lives. The Swan is one of many exercises he designed to help combat this pervasive pattern.

A healthy spine has three natural curves – in the neck (cervical spine), in the ribcage area (thoracic spine) and in the lower back (lumbar spine). The cervical and lumbar areas of the spine curve forwards, towards the front of the body, and the thoracic spine curves backwards to balance the other two. These curves should be strong yet malleable, to enable the entire spine to move with flexibility and resiliency. For example, you can't breathe deeply if your thoracic spine doesn't move as you inhale and exhale. The Swan promotes better flexibility throughout your spine.

In the mat-work exercises that precede the Swan, you've often worked lying face-up on the mat, and you've articulated your spine and pelvis by bending forwards or by lifting your legs up and in towards your torso. The sequence of Pilates mat-work exercises alternates the direction and type of the workload posed by each movement. This constant balancing of force and activity keeps all your body's muscles and joints evenly engaged – essential for the Pilates goal of uniform development.

What Is the Swan?

To perform the basic intermediate version of the Swan, you lie prone (on your front), forehead down, with your palms on the mat under your shoulders, your legs extended straight back with softly pointed toes. You centre your body's strength and balance by engaging your scoop, then inhale and press your hands into the mat as you lift your head, shoulders, chest and then stomach off the mat into a backward curl. As you exhale, you slowly lower your body back to the mat, to your starting position. During the exercise, you pay special attention to the articulation of your vertebrae, as you slowly and precisely raise and lower your upper body.

In order to engage your abdominals for performing the Swan correctly and safely, you first must knead, massage and stretch your back muscles with the forward spine and hip-flexing exercises that precede it in the mat-work series. The Swan is safe to do only after your body is well prepared in this fashion.

What the Swan Does

The spine is the body's central support system, and it depends upon the strong, active support of the Powerhouse, shoulder and thigh muscles to maintain its erect, balanced position. Because this support network is relatively complex, it's prone to a number of problems that can ruin or misalign the body's posture and balance. A misaligned pelvis – one rotated too far forwards or backwards – can lead to some common spine and posture problems. When your pelvis is rotated too far forwards, it leads to tightness in the overrounded shoulders and sunken chest, and in the overarched lower back and front of the hips. This position results in a protruding stomach and overstretched upper-back, gluteal and hamstring muscles. You stand awkwardly, your head juts forwards, you breathe shallowly and you move with greater effort and less agility.

Rotate your hips too far backwards, tucking under, and you set yourself up for a whole new set of problems. You develop tight hamstrings, gluteals and inner thighs, compounded by overstretched hip flexors and lumbar muscles and tight, weak abdominals. This scenario can result in sciatica problems, herniated discs and general mid-back and neck stress.

Good pelvic position requires strong abdominal muscles, and the Swan strengthens your abdominal muscles even as it increases their resiliency. At the same time, the Swan stretches your hip flexor and thigh muscles, relieving tightness and enabling your abdominals to engage and fire effectively – essential for maintaining proper pelvic placement and an erect, powerful posture. The Swan promotes a healthy, well-balanced pelvis; a strong, flexible spine; and uniform body strength for a strong, effective central support system.

Here are just some of the ways the Swan earns its place in the Pilates mat-work series:

· It extends your spine to decompress and articulate the vertebrae and to counter the effects of the generally forward-bending motions of your lifestyle.
· It stretches and expands your chest for deeper, healthier breathing.
· It strengthens and stretches the Powerhouse, creating a more resilient, shock-absorbing corset of midsection muscles.
· It strengthens back, neck and shoulder muscles and makes these muscle groups more flexible and resilient.
· It stabilizes the shoulder girdle and integrates it to the Powerhouse.
· It strengthens your inner thighs, pelvic floor muscles, hamstrings and gluteals.
· It stretches tight abdominals, quadriceps and hip flexor muscles.

You've seen how many Pilates spine exercises (such as the Saw) help stimulate the nervous system by rotating the spinal column and thus massaging the nerves of the spinal cord. Because the Swan moves your spine in a unique way, it provides an entirely different and valuable type of spinal cord massage.

In addition to all these benefits, the stretching and decompressing action of the Swan boosts your circulation, which in turn sends more life-giving oxygen surging throughout your body, nourishing all your joints, muscles and organs.

Tips and Precautions for Doing the Swan

Like all Pilates exercises, the Swan requires that you keep the Pilates guiding principle of concentration and awareness before you at all times. Because you're bending your body's central support structure, each moment in this exercise matters. To get the most from the basic intermediate Swan, keep these tips and precautions in mind:

· The Swan shouldn't cause pain. Arch your spine only as far as you can without any compression or strain in your shoulders, neck or lower back.
· Always keep your abdominal scoop powerfully engaged to stabilize and support your body and guide it surely and safely through the spine extensions in the Swan.
· Keep your shoulder girdle stable and wide as your palms press the mat – don't let your chest sink down, and don't allow your shoulders to pull back off your ribcage or rise up towards the back of your head. Stabilizing your shoulder girdle helps to engage your abdominals more effectively.
· Keep your elbows pulled in close to your waist and reaching backwards.
· Allow your lumbar spine and sacrum to gently arch in harmony with the rest of your spine.
· Don't overtighten your gluteals or tuck your pelvis under.
· Keep your legs parallel – don't allow them to turn out at the hips.
· Stretch your hamstrings towards the ceiling to keep knees straight.

The Basic Swan Exercise

To transition from the Saw to the Swan, exhale as you bring your legs together in front of you, keeping them straight and your toes softly pointed. Squeeze your legs together and inhale as you sweep them around behind you and roll forwards to lie on your belly. Exhale, scooping deeply, as you place your palms flat on the mat under your shoulders and your forehead on the mat (see FIGURE 17-1). Then, follow these steps to do the Swan:

1. Inhale slowly as you engage your scoop by drawing your stomach in and up along the front of your spine. Move your gaze forwards along the mat, lift your eyes and chin, and gently arch your neck and then your upper back (see FIGURE 17-2). Begin to press your palms into the mat, as you continue to sweep your gaze up the wall in front of you as each vertebra rises from the mat, lifting your ribs and stomach (maybe even the top of your pelvis) off the mat. Continue to inhale until you've arched your back as far as you can without any compression or strain in your lower back, shoulders or neck (see FIGURE 17-3). Remember to keep your scoop, as if you're trying to touch the front of your spine with your abdominal muscles.

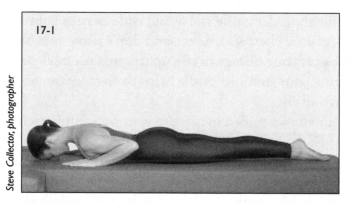

17-1

Steve Collector, photographer

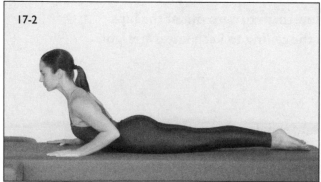

17-2

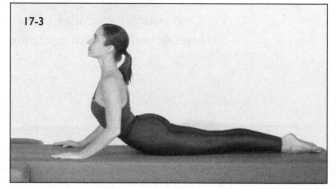

17-3

2. Squeeze your abdominal corset tighter and tighter and slowly exhale as you lower first your pelvis, then your scooped abdomen and finally your chest and head back towards your starting position. As your body lowers, stretch out along the mat to make your spine longer and more decompressed than when you started.
3. Repeat steps 1 and 2 three or four more times.

Things to Remember as You Do the Swan

When you finish the Swan, you should feel tall, energized and refreshed. If you experienced any problems as you worked through this exercise, here are some ideas that might help your performance:

· Use your stomach and back muscles to help lift your spine from the mat – don't just push up with your arms. Imagine yourself as the figurehead on the prow of a boat.
· Create a uniform curve in your arching back and neck. Don't overarch your lower back or neck to gain altitude with the Swan. Use a mirror to help you achieve this.
· Use your breath and flowing natural movement to ease your body in and out of the powerful curve of this exercise, and to reduce unnecessary tension and effort.
· Be aware of the placement and position of your entire body while you concentrate on articulating your spine vertebra by vertebra.
· Time your breathing so that your lungs inhale to their fullest capacity at the very top of your arching movement, and so that you finish exhaling (squeezing that last atom of air from your lungs) when your forehead touches the mat at the end of each repetition.
· Use the oppositional energy of your tightly squeezed legs to stretch away from your scooped stomach and lengthened spine.
· To properly engage and elongate your body's muscles and joints when you begin the Swan, imagine that your spine is a spring being stretched away from your squeezing inner thighs.

The following visualization will help you train your body's movements to get the safest, most effective extension of your spine. Imagine you're a snake lying under a big round boulder, and you decide to sneak out from under the rock to get some sun. Leading with your eyes, you stretch your head, neck and spine up along the curving underside of the boulder as you move your body forwards, up and around it. Don't push the boulder backwards, but use your stomach muscles and hands to gently pull your body forwards, up and along that broad upward curve. The lower part of your body – your legs – is held under the boulder, creating a long, deep stretch in your body as you reach towards the warmth of the sun, which touches your face, shoulders and chest.

Beginner's Modifications for the Swan

Because the Swan requires you to move your spine in a wholly new way, this exercise is likely to be quite challenging when you first begin your Pilates practice. You may have a tendency to overemphasize the arch of your neck and lower back as you curve up, because those areas of your spine naturally curve in the same direction as the Swan movement. You need to stabilize your pelvis and your shoulder girdle, and engage your abdominals powerfully to overcome that tendency. Each preceding exercise has helped you strengthen and prepare these muscles and joints for the important work of the Swan – that's why the Swan comes at this later stage of the mat-work series.

At this point in your Pilates practice, you've learned to read your body more effectively. As you choose and use modifications for the Swan, carefully assess what physical tightness, weakness or imbalance you might need to compensate for with your early modifications. As your body develops, continue assessing and altering modifications to keep the Swan both challenging and safe.

If you tend to bend too much in your lower back, creating undue compression or strain, you can modify the Swan in several ways:

· Limit your spine extension to your head, neck and upper back, and be sure to maintain a powerful scoop (to refresh your memory, see the sections on the Pilates scoop in Chapters 7 and 8).
· Place a folded towel under your hipbones to assist in keeping your lower back long.

- Move your hands a few centimetres forward on the mat to help you better flex your upper thoracic area and to discourage you from pushing your spine backwards by bending your lower back too soon.
- Working on an official Pilates mat (or folded blankets approximately 10cm/4in thick placed over a non-skid surface), you can hang your toes or your whole foot off the mat. Another strategy is to move your body down the mat until your hip joints reach the edge so that your pelvis rests on the mat and your thighs extend off the mat with knees on the floor. These positions release tight hip flexor and ankle muscles that may be inhibiting spinal extension or abdominal support, so it promotes better articulation of the upper spine.
- Working on the 10cm/4in mat, you can slide your body forwards until your head, shoulders and upper ribcage are off the mat, hands on the floor. This position can facilitate better movement in your thoracic spine and reduce an excessive lumbar curve.

If you still struggle with a tendency to crunch your neck, shoulders or lower back, try the Swan sitting up. Use a mirror to check the curve of your body, and make sure it's uniform from the crown of your head through your coccyx. Your stomach should remain tautly scooped to support your body in this smooth, uniform curve.

If your lower back, hips or shoulders are tight, begin the Swan in a kneeling position to help you focus on articulating your upper spine. Here's how to do it:

1. Kneel on the mat and sit lightly on your heels, with your legs folded under you, toes gently pointed.
2. Raise your hands as high as your ears, elbows bent and palms facing forward, like a mime touching an imaginary wall.
3. Inhale, scooping your stomach as you pull your shoulder blades down, and then press them forwards toward the front of your body, lifting your chest to the ceiling; keep your eyes and face lifted upward to where the wall and ceiling meet. Pull your elbows wide, without moving your hands to increase your upper-back curve and shoulder girdle stability (see FIGURE 17-4).

4. Exhale by tightening your corset of abdominal muscles to pull your ribs down and straighten your spine to return to the starting position.

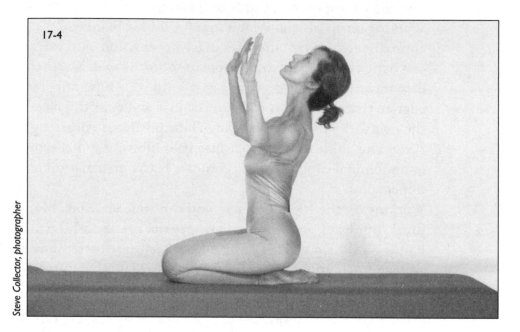

17-4

Steve Collector, photographer

Progressing Beyond the Beginner's Level

As your strength and skills increase, use any of the following modifications to progress towards the basic version:

· Begin the exercise by pulling your shoulder blades down the back of your ribcage and pulling gently backwards with your palms (just pull back on the mat, don't actually move your hands) – this action helps to stabilize your shoulder girdle. As your spine rises, continue the downward movement of your shoulder blades, and then feel the blades gently pushing forwards through your body, as if your shoulder blades were hands pushing your chest forwards and up. Allow your neck to rise easily up out of this lift, without strain.

· Use the above modification, but rise only partially from the mat, then pause. Lighten the weight you're supporting with your hands by shifting more support to your abdomen and back, then feel your upper back muscles strengthen. Maintain this feeling in your back – as well as your scoop – as you lower your body to the starting position.

· Repeat the partial rise from the mat (described in the preceding list of modifications), then lift your hands completely off the mat a little so that they're no longer supporting any weight; hold this position for one breath. This modification strengthens your upper back and abdominals even more. Place your hands back on the mat, but more lightly than before, and use your back and abdominal strength to lower yourself to your starting position.

When practising modifications for the Swan, be sure to maintain a strong, powerful scoop and don't push your stomach into the mat. You want your abdominal muscles to play a leading role in supporting your body's weight, so maintain concentration on the way you engage and use those muscles.

Here's another visualization that can help you learn to master the Swan by helping to articulate your body's curve more slowly and gently as it relieves tension and compression in your shoulders and spine.

Imagine that your eyes are following the movements of a ladybird as it travels away from you, across the mat and floor, and up the wall in front of you. When your body is arched upwards as far as you can take it today, imagine that the ladybird reverses its path; again, follow its movements as it crawls back down the wall and towards you.

The Ultimate Version of the Swan

The Swan Dive I and the Swan Dive II are advanced versions of the Swan. These exercises teach your body new skills, lifting your legs from the mat and rocking. But before you move to those advanced versions, try this intermediate exercise:

1. Lie facing down on the mat as in your original Swan starting position, forehead down and palms flat on the mat under your

shoulders, legs squeezed together and stretching back and away from your scooped stomach.

2. Concentrate on your left leg; as you exhale, stretch and straighten your left leg (especially the knee), and stretch the whole leg away from you along the mat until it begins to rise only a couple of centimetres. Lengthening the leg is more important than lifting it high off the mat. Feel the stretch extending from your stomach, across the front of your hip and down the front of your thigh. Your hamstrings are working powerfully to extend your hip and lift your leg; don't bend your knee! Use a mirror to make sure your knee is straight. Keep both hipbones on the mat, and don't tuck.

3. Inhale as you continue to stretch your leg – reaching it as far as possible away from you – and lightly lower it to the mat.

4. Repeat steps 2 and 3 with the right leg, doing three sets of this exercise with alternate legs.

5. Next, lift both legs simultaneously, and repeat three times. Remember: long is more important than high.

6. Exhale as you scoop your stomach deep into your spine to lift your hips off the mat and set them back on your heels. Rest in this position for several breaths to stretch and release your spine (especially the lumbar area).

The Swan Dive I

The Swan Dive I is a great advanced-level version of the Swan. To begin, lie face-down on the mat in your original Swan starting position, forehead down and palms flat on the mat under your shoulders, legs squeezed together and stretched away from your scooped stomach. Then follow these steps:

1. Inhale slowly as you deepen your scoop (imagine that the entire length of your spine is a spring being stretched away from your squeezing inner thighs), and move your gaze forwards along the mat, lifting your eyes and chin, gently arching your neck and then upper back.

   Begin to press your palms into the mat and allow your gaze to continue rising up the wall in front of you as you slowly lift your spine (vertebra by vertebra), your ribs, your stomach and possibly even the top of your pelvis off the mat. Continue to inhale until you've arched your back as far as you can without any compression or strain in your lower back, shoulders or neck. Keep your abdominals scooped.

2. Lift your palms slightly from the mat as you exhale and rock forwards onto your ribcage. Use your hamstrings to stretch your legs long and away from you and up towards the ceiling. Keep your legs straight and as close together as possible.

3. Inhale as you press your palms back into the mat and push your torso up again; your legs will return to the mat.

4. Repeat steps 2 and 3 three more times (this is a fairly brisk movement), then sit back for a few moments in the rest position.

With each repetition of the Swan Dive I, you will be able to arch your spine further and straighten your elbows and knees more. Be sure to keep your shoulder blades down and your stomach scooped. Use oppositional energy to stretch your squeezing inner thighs away from your taut stomach, so you don't tuck or grip your gluteals.

Swan Dive II

When you've mastered the basic intermediate version of the Swan and the Swan Dive I, you no longer need your arms to push your torso up off the mat and you have ample control of your Powerhouse, pelvis and shoulder girdle. Now, you're ready to try this version:

1. Repeat step 1 of the Swan Dive I.

2. Slide your palms forwards and away from you, then turn your palms up as you exhale and rock forwards onto your ribcage. Use your hamstrings to reach both your legs long and away from you and up towards the ceiling. Keep your shoulder blades down and your legs close together and as straight as possible (see FIGURE 17-5).

3. Inhale as you lift your body up in a backward rocking motion, to rise up on your pelvis (see FIGURE 17-6). To help carry your body into this position, imagine you're tossing a big beach ball behind you over your head with both hands. Keep your shoulder blades down.

4. Continue exhaling and inhaling as you rock forwards and backwards, like a rocking chair, five times. Sit back into the rest position.

As you perform the Swan Dive II, use the guiding principle of oppositional energy to lengthen and decompress your spine and stretch your abdominals like a taut elastic band. As you rock forward, imagine that you're stretching your body and arms to catch a beach ball before it hits the ground; as you rock back, imagine throwing a beach ball even further behind you each time.

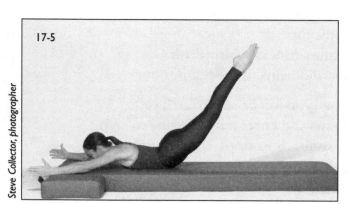
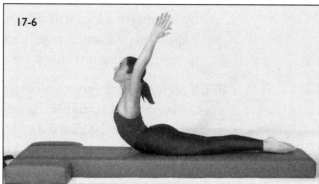

Steve Collector, photographer

17-5

17-6

Using the Swan in Other Movements

As the Swan lengthens, aligns and balances your body, it strengthens your back, hips and abdominal muscles and stretches your shoulders, chest and thighs. All of these improvements help you breathe more deeply, walk more energetically and move with greater ease, balance and stability – you are more in sync with the waterfall of gravity.

Beyond the benefits to daily movements and activities, the unique spine-extending capabilities of the Swan are of great use to athletes. Gymnasts need the Swan's benefit of a long, flexible spine to do a back layout; divers use this benefit to arch backwards as they jackknife off the diving platform. Climbers need a strong, flexible spine to reach for overhanging holds, and jumpers and vaulters depend on the spine's resilience and length to make a high jump or clear a pole. Bowlers in cricket, golfers, tennis players and fly fishermen all employ the Swan's backbending skill (in combination with other Pilates skills, such as the spinal twisting you learned in Chapter 16).

Many of the Pilates equipment exercises increase spinal extension, and therefore take the skills you learn in the Swan to the next level. You can do versions of the Swan on a variety of Pilates equipment, including the Universal Reformer, the Trapeze Table, the Chair and the High Barrel. Each piece of equipment supports the exercise in different ways, enabling students to access areas of their body that are difficult to reach without additional aid.

Pilates Reformer exercises that call upon your ability to extend your spine in a backward motion include the High Bridge, Pull Straps and T, Tree, Thigh Stretch with Arch, Semicircle, Backbend, Back Headstands and Knee Stretches with Arch. On the Trapeze Table, you'll bend backwards when you perform the Cat with the Push Through Bar, the Waterwheel, the Hanging Down and Up, the Squirrel and the Inversions, an exercise that challenges the skills you learn in the Swan as you hang from the top bars (see FIGURE 17-7).

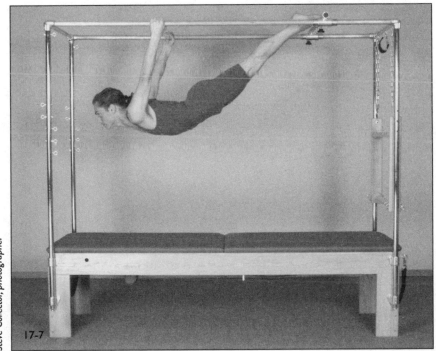

Steve Collector, photographer

17-7

'Be sure never to repeat the selected exercise(s) more than the prescribed number of times... this infraction creates muscular fatigue. There is really no need for tired muscles. Judicious selection of Contrology exercises will accomplish more for your health and bodily condition... than all else combined.'

Joseph Pilates, *Return to Life Through Contrology*

CHAPTER 18

The Side Kick I and II

The Side Kick exercises give you the opportunity to use the skills you've learned so far in a new relationship to gravity – while lying on your side. In addition, the asymmetrical nature of this exercise develops a coordination and balance unlike any preceding exercise in the mat work.

What You Need to Know about the Side Kicks

In the mat-work series, you just finished the Spine Stretch and the Saw (exercises that concentrate on spinal articulation, flexion and rotation), and then the Swan, an exercise that extends the spine. In the Side Kick exercises, your focus will return to stabilizing your spine and pelvis with a body and mind more alert, capable and resilient than it has been at any previous point in your workout. To balance on your side during this exercise, you must have greater whole-body awareness and keener concentration and control of each individual movement of your spine, pelvis and legs.

What Are the Side Kicks?

To perform the Side Kicks, you lie on one side of your body and extend your straight legs together and in front of you at a 45-degree angle from your hips. Your bottom hand supports your head, and your other hand presses into the mat in front of your chest. You stabilize your spine with your Powerhouse as you lift your top leg and sweep it forwards and backwards (with an additional pulse at either end) eight to ten times. Then you rotate your top leg outwards and kick it up towards the ceiling and then down, eight to ten times.

When you finish the Side Kicks you'll notice some dramatic changes in the way your body feels. Your hips will be freer, your stomach more supportive, and your spine more erect and stable. You'll feel tall, flexible and as graceful as a dancer.

What the Side Kicks Do

The Side Kicks are especially effective in strengthening your outer hip muscles, especially the *gluteus medius* muscle located at the top of your outer hip. The *gluteus medius* is essential for good posture, hip integrity and control.

To feel this muscle in action, try this: stand upright with legs together. Use a powerful Pilates scoop to stand as tall and erect as you can, feeling your feet rooted into the ground. Place your hands on your hips just behind your hipbones, and bend one knee forwards as you lift that foot slightly off the ground, keeping your pelvis level. Notice the tensing of the muscle on the outer hip of the standing leg. This muscle is working to keep your pelvis level and stable.

Now try to keep your hips level and centred as you walk – no swaying. This pelvic stabilization skill is essential to maintaining health in your lower back, pelvis, hips, knees and, ultimately, your whole body. The Side Kicks are the most effective exercises for building this skill.

When you add the complexity and challenge of sweeping your top leg forwards and backwards parallel to the ground while staying in sync with gravity, you begin to feel the powerful benefits this exercise has to offer. Performing the Side Kicks elevates your spirit because it shows off all your hard-won capabilities!

The Side Kicks also stretch tight leg muscles, such as your quadriceps, hip flexors, hamstrings and inner and outer thighs. These exercises are another great example of the unique Pilates paradigm, in which you work to create resilient, strong, flexible, toned tissue by strengthening and stretching your muscles simultaneously.

Working on your side in the Side Kicks gives you an opportunity to add to and refine the strength and power of your core. When you lie flat on your back or stomach, more of your body surface is pulled down by gravity. As a result, your muscles are primarily working to oppose this force as you move. When you lie on your side, less of your body is exposed to this force, and therefore you are more in sync with – rather than in opposition to – the waterfall of gravity.

Tips and Precautions
for Doing the Side Kicks

Awareness, concentration and control are all guiding principles of Pilates. These principles provide powerful safeguards when you make large, sweeping movements with your extended limbs, as you do in the Side Kicks. Keep these tips and precautions in mind as you work through these exercises:

- Keep your legs straight and slightly turned out, with your feet softly pointed.
- Move your extended leg with control, reaching and sweeping it through space. Don't swing it or allow the movement to build momentum.
- Keep your hips and shoulders stacked on top of each other and in complete alignment – as if you could drop a plumb line through them. Don't allow any twists.
- Move your leg as one unit from the hip joint; keep your knee completely straight and your leg stretched long.
- Keep your spine and pelvis stable. Don't tuck or twist.
- Use your bottom leg to stabilize and support your torso; concentrate on stretching it away from you at a 45-degree angle.
- Keep pressing the hand that is in front of your chest into the mat; use its support to centre you and enable you to work your Powerhouse and to maintain a stable ribcage.
- Experiment with the placement of the hand supporting your head to find the position that facilitates good spine, shoulder and head posture. Keep your head aligned with your neck and your gaze forwards; use a mirror to check for alignment. Monitor yourself for neck tension or strain.
- Stretch your bottom shoulder blade down your back as you stretch your elbow away. This action integrates your shoulder girdle into your core and makes you more stable.
- If you feel or hear a clunk or pop as you sweep your leg, use oppositional energy to reach your leg away from your stable pelvis and your scooped abdominals, engaging the muscles around your hip more effectively, powerfully and uniformly to decompress the hip joint.

For Side Kick I

When you're doing the Side Kick I, keep in mind these special tips and precautions:

- Keep your leg parallel to the mat as it sweeps forwards and backwards. Don't allow it to drop towards the mat as it moves forwards, or to lift towards the ceiling in the back.
- Keep your leg slightly rotated outwards as you sweep to the front and back, to engage your outer hip. Don't let your leg turn in as you move it forwards, or turn out more as you move it to the back.
- The pulsing action at the end of each movement gives your hamstrings and hip flexors more stretch as it strengthens your abdominals. Don't bounce your leg; make it travel further by 5 to 7.5cm (2 to 3in) on the pulse.

 If your torso rocks as you perform the Side Kick I, shorten your leg's range of motion. Don't sacrifice the stabilizing strength in your core for a big, high kick in any direction.

- Keep your top hip lengthened away from your ribs; don't shorten your waist.
- As you sweep the leg, practise ribcage stability, maintaining a stable, unmoving torso and shoulder girdle; don't counterbalance the sweeping motion by tilting or rocking your torso or shoulders.

For Side Kick II

Here are some special tips and precautions for Side Kick II:

- Keep your pelvis and spine stable, one hip joint stacked above the other, as you rotate your femur in your hip joint to turn out the top leg. Don't tuck, arch or twist your spine or pelvis.
- Arc your leg straight up to the ceiling without twisting your pelvis or shifting your hip. This strengthens your outer hip and deep hip rotators, and increases the range of motion of your hip joint.

· Keep your top hip lengthened away from your ribs. Don't shorten your waist.

Two Versions of the Basic Side Kick Exercise

The Side Kick I and Side Kick II are both effective exercises for building strong, flexible muscles in your Powerhouse, hips and legs, and each offers unique benefits to the body. In the beginning, you can choose to stick with one version. However, as your stamina and skills develop, you can transition from Side Kick I into Side Kick II.

Step by Step Through the Basic Side Kick I

To transition from the Swan's rest position to the Side Kick I exercise, lie on the mat on your left side, with your legs slightly turned out, stacked on top of each other, stretching straight out and together at a 45-degree angle from the front of your body. (If you have an official Pilates mat, your feet will move forwards on top of a foot box.)

Keep your toes softly pointed. Your left arm is bent and supporting your head, forming a straight line from your elbow to your coccyx. Your eyes are looking straight out in front of you with a relaxed, aligned neck. Your right arm is bent, palm pressing the mat in front of your chest. Now, follow these steps to perform the basic intermediate Side Kick I:

1. Lift your right leg a few centimetres to be hip height, and reach it long and away from you (see FIGURE 18-1). Inhale, scooping to increase the length between your ribs and your hips, and sweep your right leg forwards, parallel to the mat, until you feel a gentle stretch in your hamstring (see FIGURE 18-2).
2. Continue to inhale as you deepen your scoop and pulse your leg by reaching it several centimetres further at the end of your sweeping motion; keep the rest of your body stable and still.

3. Exhale to clinch the laces of your corset and stabilize your body as you sweep your right leg backwards, parallel to the mat; continue back until you feel a gentle stretch in the front of your abdomen, hip and thigh (see FIGURE 18-3).

4. Again, continue to exhale as you pulse your leg by reaching it 5 or 7.5cm (2 or 3in) further at the end of your sweep. Keep your stomach scooped in and up the front of your spine.

5. Repeat steps 2 to 4 for a total of eight to ten times, then finish by stacking your right leg back on top of your left.

6. Transition to Side Kick II (described in the section that follows) or turn over and repeat steps 1 through 5 of this version, using the left leg.

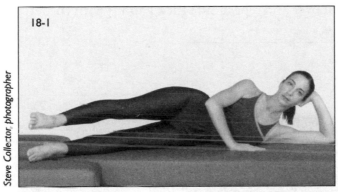

18-1

Steve Collector, photographer

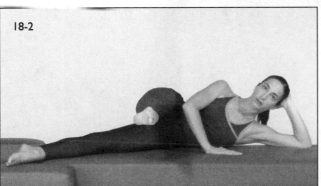

18-2

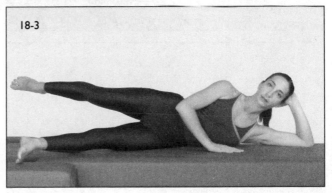

18-3

Step by Step Through the Basic Side Kick II

To transition from Side Kick I, rotate your right leg in your hip joint to turn out further, and place your right heel slightly in front of your left ankle (see FIGURE 18-4). Keep your hips stacked; don't tuck or twist. Then follow these steps:

1. Inhale to scoop your stomach in and up the front of the spine as you sweep your right leg out and away from you and up towards your ear; imagine that you're reaching your leg so far away from your hip that you touch the wall on the other side of the room and then the ceiling with your toes during this movement (see FIGURES 18-5 and 18-6). Keep your waist long and your hips stacked one on top of the other.
2. Exhale as you reach your leg even further away from you to draw the leg back down, right heel finishing in front of left foot.
3. Repeat steps 1 and 2, for a total of eight to ten times.
4. Turn over and repeat Side Kick I and II with the left leg.

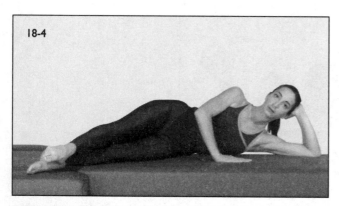

18-4

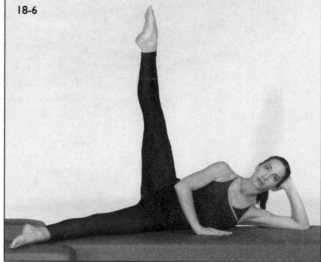

18-6

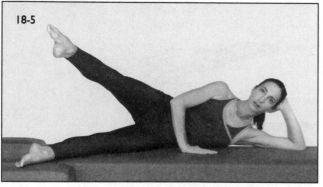

18-5

Things to Remember as You Do the Side Kicks

The Side Kick I and II are both powerful, elegant movements that require controlled, sweeping motions – you won't get the full benefit from this exercise if you swing your legs wildly. As you practise the Side Kicks, remember these guidelines to help keep your form:

- To build full-body, uniform development, be aware of your entire body as you concentrate on stabilizing your torso so you can freely move your leg in the hip joint.
- To elongate your spine and centre yourself, use oppositional energy to reach your sitz bones away from the crown of your head and to reach your working leg away from your hip or even away from your stable supporting leg.
- Press your bottom leg into the mat to further stabilize you and strengthen that hip.
- Use the forward and upward sweeping motions to help boost your inhalation and elongate your spine; use the backward and downward sweeps to propel the air out of your lungs and to decompress and stabilize your spine.
- In Side Kick I, use the pulsing motion of the leg to the front to increase the depth of your inhalation, and use the pulsing motion of the leg to the back to deepen your exhale – to wring the last atom of air out of your lungs.
- Make your leg movements swift, flowing and smooth.

Beginner's Modifications for the Side Kicks

It's a challenge to perform big, sweeping motions with an extended leg while lying on your side and anchoring the rest of the body along the mat. Your first goal for these exercises should be to maintain your stability during the movement; if that means you have to limit the movement initially, then do it – you'll still benefit from the exercises, and you'll expand your range of motion in time. Here are some suggestions for modifying the Side Kicks:

- If you feel any strain in your neck or shoulders, extend your bottom arm up along the mat in line with your spine, and rest your head on your arm (see FIGURE 18-7). You can also put a small pillow between your arm and head.
- If you can't keep your pelvis and spine stable or your legs straight, limit the range of motion of your sweeping leg as it moves to the front, back or side.
- Bend the supporting leg and move it forwards a bit to help stabilize your torso and to bring your pelvis into a neutral alignment. Press the bent leg into the mat.
- Cut the number of repetitions.

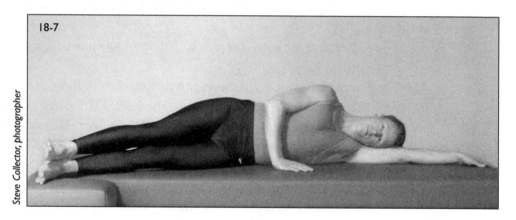

18-7

Steve Collector, photographer

The Ultimate Version of the Side Kicks

As you work with the basic intermediate or modified versions of the Side Kicks I and II, your body will develop strength, stability and flexibility. When you've achieved more uniform development, strong core stability and leg and hip flexibility, you can make these exercises more challenging with these advanced modifications:

- To further challenge your core stability, place your top arm's hand behind your head instead of anchoring it into the mat (see FIGURE 18-8). Press the back of your head gently into your cupping palms to help stabilize your shoulder girdle and give you better access to your upper abdominals. Keep your shoulder blades reaching down your back.

- In Side Kick I, flex your foot as you sweep your leg to the front, and strongly point the foot as you sweep it backwards. Create the flex by lengthening the entire back of the leg so much that it curls the foot into a flex; then maintain this length as you point.
- In Side Kick II, add a strong point of the foot as you sweep your leg up toward the ceiling and flex your foot as you squeeze the leg back down. Do this for the first four or five repetitions, then reverse the pattern of the flex and point for the last four or five reps.

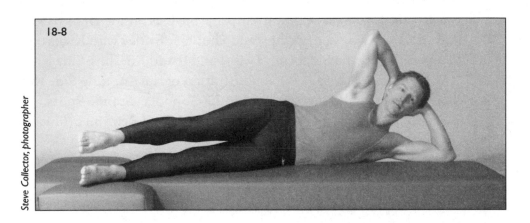

18-8

Steve Collector, photographer

Using the Side Kicks in Other Movements

The Side Kicks are powerful exercises for strengthening, stretching and balancing the pelvis and hips. You'll use this benefit every day, every time you lift one foot from the ground, whether you're rushing through busy city streets or climbing the stairs. The Side Kicks' asymmetrical training will improve your balance and keep you stable and sure on your feet as you run, walk, stretch, stoop, squat, bend and climb.

As you grow older, maintaining equilibrium is very important; falls result in thousands of broken bones every year, and many of those falls occur simply because our sense of balance can deteriorate when we lose strength and flexibility with age. Broken hips and hip replacement surgery are very common among senior citizens – thousands of older people are hospitalized for hip fractures every year. Healthy, strong hips will keep you active longer.

The core strength you will develop practising the Side Kicks should keep your body well aligned and supported above your pelvis, distributing the weight of your upper body evenly through your hips and down into your knees, ankles and arches. Dancers, gymnasts, runners, hurdlers, skaters, footballers and everyone else who depends on strong, well-balanced movements and coordination use the skills developed by the Side Kick exercises.

In the Pilates method, the Side Kicks prepare you for more advanced movements, such as Standing Straight Leg Press and Leg Press on the Floor on the Wunda or Low Chair; Side Sit-Ups on the High Barrel; Inversions, Flying Leg Springs, and Shoulder Bridge with Kicks on the Trapeze Table; and Sidebend, Twist I and II and Kneeling Side Kicks on the Mat. (See FIGURE 18-10 for an illustration of the Kneeling Side Kicks.) The Side Kicks also prepare you for the Gondola, Grande Splits, Control Arabesque and the Star on the Universal Reformer (illustrated in FIGURE 18-11).

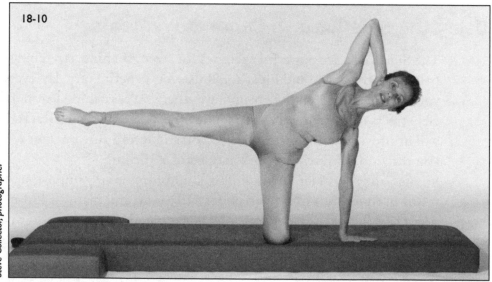

18-10

Steve Collector, photographer

'Concentrate on the correct movements each time you exercise, lest you do them improperly and thus lose all the vital benefits of their value. Correctly executed and mastered, these exercises will reflect grace and balance in your routine activities.'

Joseph Pilates, *Return to Life Through Contrology*

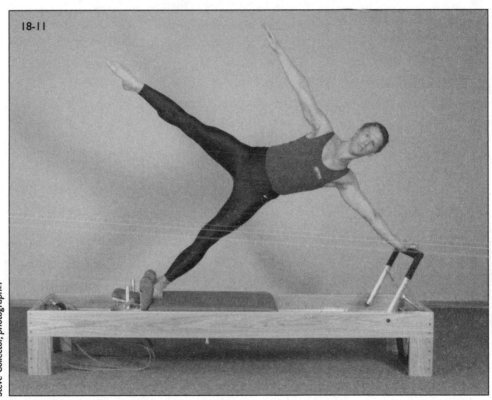

Steve Collector, photographer

CHAPTER 19
The Seal

Congratulations! You've reached the final exercise in your Pilates mat-work series. The Seal holds true to all the Pilates guiding principles and incorporates most of the fundamental movement skills, and it is also fun to do – think of it as the dessert at the end of a hard workout.

What You Need to Know about the Seal

The preceding Side Kick exercises focused on strengthening your hips and powerfully stabilizing your spine against the force of one moving leg while lying on your side. The Seal follows those exercises by returning you to a seated, symmetrical, forward-facing position that aligns you upright in the waterfall of gravity, and flexes and massages your spine in much the same way as the Rolling Like a Ball exercise. The Seal releases the hips and hip joints after the powerful, stabilizing and strengthening hip exercises that precede it.

The Seal is a demanding exercise, but because it is the last in the Pilates mat-work series, it is also a cool-down exercise. Because you perform it last, you're able to approach the Seal calmly, with the ease, strength and mental focus built throughout your workout.

What Is the Seal?

To perform the Seal exercise, you sit facing forwards on the mat, knees bent and open to the sides, heels together, gently pressing your inner thighs into your arms and vice versa, as you cup an ankle in each hand. You lift your heels and balance on your coccyx or sacrum, then inhale as you roll back to your shoulder blades, lifting your hips above your head and suspending them in this position as you clap your heels together three times. You finish the Seal by exhaling and rolling back down your spine to return to the starting balance, and clap your heels again three times.

What the Seal Does

The Seal caps your workout with a calming, centring movement; its stretching and balancing action brings your body back to its forward orientation and prepares you to stand, sit and move with coordination and control throughout the remainder of your day. Here are some other benefits of the Seal:

·   It increases blood flow along the spine.
·   It strengthens your abdominal corset, enabling you to decompress and stabilize your spine and to exhale effectively.

- It strengthens your inner thighs, pelvic floor, deep hip rotators and gluteal muscles.
- It stabilizes your shoulder girdle and integrates it into your core.
- It trains balance and coordination.
- It releases hip joint tension, and helps you learn to move the femur and pelvis independently of each other.
- The rolling motion of the Seal massages the spine to increase flexibility between the vertebrae, ribs and back muscles, increasing your breathing capacity.

What are the benefits of integrating my shoulder girdle into my core?

When your shoulder girdle is linked to the strength of your core, you supply stability and power to your shoulder and arm movements. Your Powerhouse is the essential centre of all your body's movements. When the muscles of your shoulder girdle draw strength from a strong, stable core, you support the extended movements of your arms, to prevent strain and stress injuries.

Tips and Precautions for Doing the Seal

In many ways, the Seal is similar to the Rolling Like a Ball exercise, which you learned in Chapter 12 of this book. (You may want to refer to some of these tips and precautions from that chapter.)

Here's what you should keep in mind as you perform the Seal:

- Suspend the backward roll when you reach the area between your shoulder blades. Your head and neck never touch the mat (use the principle of precise control).
- Make your rolling motion smooth and sequential; if you find yourself flopping or crashing backwards like a flat tyre instead of a round wheel, use the modifications and visualizations offered later in this chapter to practise aspects of the exercise before coordinating them into a whole.

- Keep your eyes focused on your pubic bone throughout the entire exercise. Don't throw your head back and forth in an effort to build up momentum for the rolling motion.
- To help promote a full, healthy lower-spine curl, visualize that you're reaching your sitz bones or coccyx around towards the back of your knees as you scoop your stomach in and up. This visualization strengthens your abdominals, gluteals and hamstrings, and uses the guiding principle of oppositional energy to stretch a tight lower back.
- Imagine that you're squeezing a beach ball between your knees while you roll and unroll. This squeezing motion helps you access the power of your stomach, inner thighs and pelvic floor muscles as it stretches your lower back.

If you have bone, spine or shoulder problems, such as osteoporosis, herniated or bulging vertebral discs, rods in your spine, separated shoulder, current or recent cervical injuries, severe scoliosis or spondylolisthesis, among others, the Seal could offer some potential risks of further injury. Be safe, and get your doctor's advice before attempting this exercise.

- When you curl your upper spine, keep your shoulders open and broad, your shoulder blades reaching down your back and your elbows pressing into your inner thighs. Don't allow your shoulders to scrunch up towards your ears or forwards into your chest.
- Keep elbows long, but not locked. Don't pull your feet towards you.
- Try to roll evenly down the middle of your spine, as if you were rolling along a channel or a railway track. Your natural tendency may be to roll towards one side of your spine, so pay careful attention and correct any side preferences. You can steer with your abdominals by accentuating the strength or length on one side or the other.
- Experiment to find your balanced sitting position. Depending upon your lower-back flexibility and core strength, you may need to adjust your pelvic position, either by moving slightly forwards onto your coccyx or slightly backwards onto your sacrum.

·   Gently press your inner thighs against your arms and vice versa. This stabilizes your balance and strengthens the muscles of your inner thighs, pelvic floor, shoulder girdle and Powerhouse.

·   Stabilize your entire body in its curl shape and roll the whole shape without changing it. Imagine you're inside a ball and conform your shape to its inside curl as you roll evenly back and forth. Don't pull on your feet to move.

·   Remember the wave image and curl your pelvis over your upper abs as you roll backwards; conversely, curl your upper abs over your pelvis as you roll forwards. Don't strain your neck and head; avoid hunching your shoulders.

The Basic Seal Exercise

The Seal is a centring, calming exercise designed to wrap up your workout and prepare you to move out into the demands of your day. And, as you've found with most other exercises in the Pilates mat-work series, you can make the Seal a bit easier – or more challenging – to fit your current capabilities and fitness needs.

The steps in the following section describe the basic intermediate Seal exercise. Later sections describe beginning and advanced modifications. Use these modifications as appropriate for your experience and fitness level. Keep the Seal safe, challenging and fun.

Step by Step Through the Basic Seal

To transition from the Side Kicks to the Seal, pull your stomach in as you inhale and scoop deeply to come to a sitting position, facing the front end of your mat. Exhale as you bend your knees to the sides, bringing your heels together, and curl your spine up and forwards.

Inhale as you slide your hands between your legs and under your heels to cup your outer ankles. Exhale to integrate your core, gently pressing your inner thighs to your arms and vice versa, as you balance on your coccyx, lifting your feet 7.5 or 10cm (3 or 4in) from the mat (see FIGURE 19-1). Then follow these steps:

1. Inhale and deeply scoop your abs as you roll backwards (exactly in imitation of a wheel) onto the area between your shoulder blades. Your hips are curled up and over you, and your feet are behind your head (see FIGURES 19-2 and 19-3).

2. Continue to inhale as you suspend your movement there and gently clap your heels together three times, moving your entire leg freely in your hip joint.

3. Clinch your corset to expel the air, and to propel yourself forwards to your starting position, balanced on your coccyx or sacrum.

4. Continue to exhale as you suspend your movement there and gently clap your heels together three times, once again, moving your entire leg freely in your hip joint.

Repeat steps 1 to 4 six to eight times. With each repetition, increase your spinal flexibility, hip freedom, balance, control and coordination.

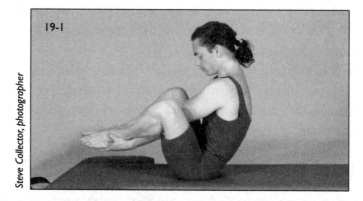

19-1

Steve Collector, photographer

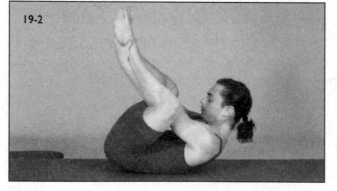

19-2

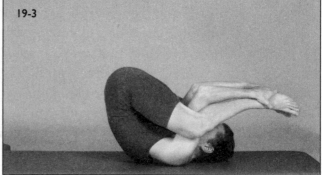

19-3

Things to Remember as You Do the Seal

Though its movements are calm and controlled, be aware of the workout this exercise gives your body throughout each repetition. Here are some guidelines to aid you in your practice of the Seal:

· Time your inhalations and exhalations to culminate with the third clap in each body position. (If necessary, review the Pilates breathing sections in Chapters 7 and 8.)

· Use the power and depth of your inhalation to elongate your spine and inflate your lungs and ribs, increasing the stretch and massage of your back muscles.

· Use the force of your exhalation to propel you forwards to your sitting position; conversely, use the rolling action to force the air out of your lungs.

· When you clap your heels, move your whole leg from the hip joint, not just your feet or ankles.

· When you return to the sitting position, you may find it difficult to balance or control your pelvis. Engage all the muscles around your pelvis – abdominals, inner thighs, hamstrings, gluteals and the pelvic floor – to stabilize yourself. Don't rock your pelvis back and forth on your sitz bones.

· To keep your movements controlled, smooth and regular, scoop your stomach in and up, squeezing an imaginary beach ball between your knees and keeping your elbows long, and gently pressing your inner thighs as you roll.

· Promote the free movement of your hip by supporting the weight of your legs with your hands, and by moving your legs with your inner thighs to clap. Increase your hips' freedom by controlling the lift and suspension of your spine with your abdominals, not your hip flexors.

· Use precise control to suspend and balance your body as you clap your heels with an even rhythm.

· Increase the fullness and power of your breath with each repetition.

· Press your arms into your inner thighs and vice versa to stabilize your shoulder girdle. Don't hunch or round your shoulders in towards your chest.

Visualization is an important key to finding and maintaining the proper shape as you roll in this exercise. You can constantly build upon the principle of oppositional energy by imagining that your sitz bones and head are reaching in opposite directions around a big beach ball. Or imagine you're inside a ball and conform your shape to its interior curves as you roll.

Beginner's Modifications for the Seal

If you have trouble with the basic intermediate version of the Seal, you can modify the exercise to make it more accessible for beginner-level skills. The easiest way to modify the Seal is simply to eliminate certain parts of the exercise – for example, the rolling or the clapping. Dropping these parts of the Seal will enable you to focus on developing the fundamental skills: building your scoop, stabilizing your pelvis and shoulder girdle, decompressing and uniformly curling your spine and using your Powerhouse.

Here are some beginning modifications for the Seal:

· Practise only the balance part of the exercise, eliminating the rolling and the claps. Balance on your coccyx or sacrum, hands cupping your heels a few centimetres off the floor. Work on using your scoop and the muscles surrounding your pelvis and shoulder girdle to curl your spine and stabilize this position while breathing. Use visualizations described in the previous section to build your control, spinal flexibility and core strength. When your skills progress, add the claps to this balance shape.

· Do the basic intermediate version of the Seal, but eliminate the clapping portion and practise only the roll back and forth.

· If you've eliminated the clapping portion of the Seal, add it back in slowly as your skills build by clapping only during the balanced sitting position and beginning with one or two claps instead of three.

· When you've achieved enough uniform development to roll smoothly and enough core power to suspend your hips above your head for a moment, begin to add the claps there, too – first one, then two, then finally all three.

- If you're struggling with tightness that makes cupping your heels difficult, simply hold the front of your shins above your ankles with your arms still on the inside of your legs. Gently press your inner thighs against your arms to help strengthen your muscles and stabilize your balance.
- Cut repetitions, as necessary.

If you tend to roll to one side or the other during the Seal, the exercise is simply pointing out imbalances in your body's structure and development. Use these clues to learn where you need to focus special attention and apply that newfound knowledge during your Pilates workout. Your instructor can help you determine where the imbalances exist; continued Pilates practice will work to eliminate them.

The Ultimate Version of the Seal

As you achieve a more uniformly articulate and strong spine and a more integrated and controlled Powerhouse, increase the challenge of the Seal. With practice, you'll develop your ability to increase and stabilize the powerful curl of your spine and hips as you roll; your feet will get closer to the floor in the overhead position, hovering around 7.5cm (3in) above the mat as you do the claps. Coordinate your breathing so that the length and depth of your inhalation supports you through the backward roll and suspends you as you clap, and the force of your exhalation squeezes your corset and deeply integrates your Powerhouse all the way through the rolling forwards and the claps.

Using the Seal in Other Movements

As with all Pilates exercises, the Seal massages, decompresses and articulates your spine and promotes body/mind integration and whole-body health. Now you can bend, stretch, breathe and think better. The Seal strengthens your Powerhouse and stabilizes your shoulder girdle and pelvis, so you can stand longer and more comfortably and lift, push, pull, climb, twist and kick with self-assurance. This exercise also trains your mental awareness and muscle coordination to improve your balance – to step confidently off the kerb or over a rock on a mountain path.

Athletes, divers, gymnasts and skateboarders depend upon strong flexible spines, powerful core strength, good balance and steady coordination every time they flip or fly through the air. Any weakness or imbalance could result in a dangerous injury, so these athletes work to cultivate the very physical qualities the Seal is designed to develop. And you needn't be an aerial artist to benefit from the Seal; yoga asanas (positions) require the same – or even higher – levels of flexibility, strength and balance (see FIGURE 19-4, which illustrates the yoga pose of Bhujapidasana).

The skills developed by practising the Seal will also enable you to eventually perform some very exciting advanced Pilates exercises. Some examples include the Squirrel and Inversions on the Trapeze Table, in which you hang upside down from the top canopy and curl and uncurl your body, while suspending your pelvis above your head. The Seal

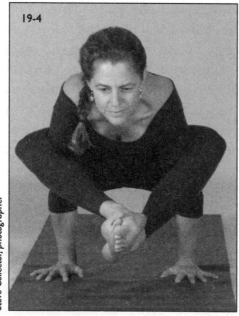

Steve Collector, photographer

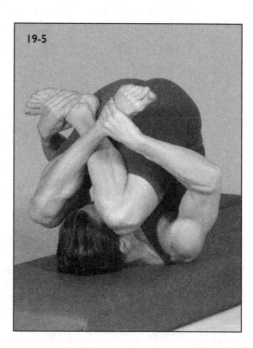

prepares you for the Short and Long Spine exercises, and the more advanced Control Arabesque on the Universal Reformer, in which you somersault off the equipment and land standing on one leg. You'll also use the skills you develop with the Seal when you perform the Crab on the Mat, in which your body curls into an even tighter ball that you must stabilize and suspend as you switch your legs (see FIGURE 19-5).

Finishing Your Mat-Work Session

You finish the ultimate version of the Seal by returning to a standing position, feeling rejuvenated and confident. To arrive at a standing position, you remove your hands from your ankles and reach forwards with straight arms, one hand on top of the other, as you exhale on the last forward roll. Cross your ankles and step onto your feet. Use your legs to push away from the floor and your Powerhouse to lift your body up and away from that push.

As you finish your first workout, congratulate yourself that you've begun to transform your body and mind. Even completing a single workout will move you closer to your Pilates goals. Each passage through the mat-work series gains you more mastery over the fundamental skills and guiding principles of the Pilates method.

As you move into an upright, balanced stance, call on all your newly developed understanding of the Pilates guiding principles in this final movement; reinforce your balanced, elongated stance with the power of oppositional energy, mental awareness and concentration, precise control, flowing natural movement, Pilates breathing and centring. Carry those principles with you as you move forwards, out of the door – and into the rest of your life.

CHAPTER 20

The Role of Pilates in Rehabilitation

Regeneration, not degeneration – that's what the Pilates method of body conditioning is all about. In fact, regeneration is essential for physical rehabilitation. Pilates is an effective method for repairing injuries and overcoming the effects of physical trauma or imbalance as it helps you regenerate your body's tissues and retrain your movements for a strong, healthy, balanced body.

Physical Rehabilitation and Pilates

When Joseph Pilates was developing his first exercises and exercise machines during World War I, the field of physical therapy was in its infancy. Today, physical rehabilitation encompasses a wide range of therapies, and Pilates is certainly among them, prescribed by many doctors and other medical professionals to relieve pain, speed recovery from surgery or injuries, aid recovery from stroke and other neurological events, and even to avoid surgical procedures. As both movement education and fitness training, Pilates is an invaluable tool for improving the general health of those suffering from chronic illnesses and systemic disabilities.

Pilates instructors aren't trained medical professionals; however, many physical therapists are now getting their Pilates certificates. Physical therapists should be trained by an approved school of physical therapy and be licensed or registered by an appropriate body.

As many doctors and physical rehabilitation specialists know, regular Pilates practice is an important tool for regaining strength, flexibility, muscle tone and overall endurance after an illness or injury, and it can help overcome some limiting disabilities. This isn't to suggest that you can buy an exercise mat and throw away your walker, but with the correct instruction and a doctor's supervision, practising Pilates can help you restore and repattern movement, reduce acute and chronic pain, recover movement after surgery and protect injured joints and muscles from further damage or reinjury.

Adjusting Your Pilates Programme

When used for rehabilitation, Pilates exercises can be modified into very simple, small, gentle movements. In time, as the student's strength and mobility build, the instructor can slowly and carefully increase the intensity of the Pilates workout until the student achieves full range of motion, stability and strength.

If you're involved in physical therapy, it's advisable that your Pilates instructor communicate with your doctor to coordinate the best rehabilitation programme for you. If you're working on Pilates at home and are currently undergoing physical therapy, make sure you have a talk with your physical therapist and your general practitioner about your Pilates programme.

Prevention of Injuries

In addition to its recovery benefits, Pilates also prevents some joint and muscle injuries. Joseph Pilates believed that the way we stand, walk and move could create stress injuries in our muscles and joints. If you have a weak muscle set, you might favour that set in your movements, and in doing so, put extra strain on other muscle groups in your body. For example, if you have joints with limited mobility, you might overwork other joints to take on the extra range your stiff joints can't bear. All this compensation can cause long-term serious damage to your body.

Because it's a whole-body workout designed to uniformly develop the body, Pilates is an excellent method of strengthening weak joints and muscles, lengthening tight tendons and muscles and balancing muscular force around the joints to prevent these compensation injuries.

Remember that the Pilates method operates on the principle that every muscle helps strengthen every other muscle. By working towards a balanced body with uniform muscle development, students can repair weakened muscles and joints, and prevent ongoing damage caused by improper posture and unbalanced movement.

The Many Therapeutic Benefits of Pilates

Pilates has been used to treat people with complications from knee, ankle, shoulder cuff, spine and hip injuries, whiplash, post-polio syndrome, car accidents, spina bifida, stroke and TMJ (temporomandibular joint) disorders, among other conditions. And those preparing for or recovering from surgeries have found the Pilates method effective in shortening their period of recovery.

Pilates is also an effective way to recover from the effects of everyday stress, strain and tension. For example, regular Pilates sessions relieve strained muscles in the neck, back and shoulders. The strengthening, posture-building impact of regular Pilates workouts actually helps your body ward off future strain as well. In addition, the mind/body unity that's such an essential ingredient of the Pilates method calms and centres you, leaving you feeling rejuvenated and relaxed.

Pilates tones muscles and balances muscular forces at the joint, and it stimulates circulation by teaching you how to achieve deep, healthy breathing, proper muscular flexibility, full joint range of movement and correct alignment.

Many people, such as the Pilates master teachers Romana Kryzanowska, Ron Fletcher and Kathy Grant, have used Pilates to avoid back or knee surgery. Pilates equipment gently and safely guides injured bodies through precise movement – a technique that works to repattern ineffective, often destructive, movement habits. Pilates is designed to strengthen weak tissue, stretch tight muscles, balance asymmetries and generally give you back the natural health you were born with.

Pregnant women have found that the Pilates method helps them develop good breath control, carry their pregnancy more comfortably and strengthen their bodies for a smoother delivery and a faster return to their pre-pregnancy body shape, stability and fitness. And Pilates is unparalleled as a postpartum fitness regime.

Pilates is particularly effective as a method for rehabilitating spine injuries. The Pilates method of body conditioning strengthens, lengthens and balances musculature around the spine, as it aligns and decompresses injured vertebrae, helping to relieve nerve and disc pressure. This decompression facilitates and stimulates healthy circulation to the damaged spinal tissue. Spinal issues such as herniated or degenerated discs, sciatica, unstable sacroiliac joints, scoliosis, arthritis, spondylolisthesis, spondylosis and spondylolysis have been successfully helped through the Pilates method.

Pilates is an effective therapy for treating a number of joint and muscle problems as well, including torn ligaments, dislocations, bursitis, tendonitis, joint replacements and separations, the effects of whiplash, carpal tunnel syndrome, thoracic outlet syndrome and piriformis syndrome. Many people have found relief from the effects of head injury and complications related to car accidents through regular Pilates practice as well.

Case Studies in Pilates Rehabilitation

To better understand the ways that Pilates can help rehabilitate injuries and overcome the effects of illness and disease, take a moment to read through a few case studies. These individuals (all names have been changed) received treatment at The Pilates Centre in Boulder, Colorado, USA, and their experiences can serve to illustrate how Pilates helps individuals return to health through regular treatment and practice in the Pilates method of body conditioning.

Pilates Helps Eliminate Lower-Back Pain

Jane came to The Pilates Centre complaining of terrible lower-back pain. She was distraught, frustrated and feeling hopeless after having seen many therapists over many years, with no beneficial results. The Centre's instructors discussed her history and evaluated her movement as she stood, walked, sat and lay down. The instructors then taught her the first several Pilates fundamental skills mini-exercises (see Chapter 8). They quickly discovered that she was unable to stabilize her lumbar spine and pelvis with her abdominals, and consequently overused her lower back muscles to such an extreme degree that movement was actually causing injury. She also exhibited asymmetrical muscle firing patterns, causing her to compress one side of her spine more than the other as she lifted one leg. Even a simple abdominal scoop or a knee fold was so painful it brought her to tears.

Using Pilates, Jane began the process of achieving uniform development in her body. Through modifications of the classic Pilates exercises, instructors taught her to be aware of her unconscious, improper movement patterns and how to move effectively, so that she could begin to strengthen the muscles that were weak and underdeveloped, and to relax those that she was overusing.

When the pain in her lower back subsided, Jane's instructors broadened the scope of their teaching focus to address other related issues, including incorrect curvature of her thoracic spine; joint pain in her knees, shoulders and elbows; and even osteoporosis. Her lack of abdominal support was contributing to all of these issues. As she strengthened her Powerhouse, the healthy natural curves of her spine re-established themselves, her lumbar vertebrae became decompressed and more flexible, her thoracic spine became more erect and aligned and her shoulders more open. Here's what Jane had to say about her experience:

> Ten years ago a neurosurgeon said that I was borderline for surgery, and that I'd never be able to do any exercise other than walking and, maybe, swimming. I was 46 at that time. However, because of studying Pilates, I now ski, backpack, scuba dive, lift weights, swim, do yoga and go dancing. The neurosurgeon was a kind man, but just didn't know much about therapeutic exercise for backs. I think sometimes about going back and showing him what I can do – with no trace of the limitations that he saw.

Pilates Eliminates Bad Posture and Movement Patterns

Carol came to The Pilates Centre for general fitness and to counteract the detrimental effects of her job. Carol's complaint is frequently heard:

> I am a systems administrator who hovers over computers all day. My life is hectic and busy. I visualize myself as a person whose head protrudes about six inches in front of me. (Surely that helps me to move quicker, right?) Pilates brings everything into perspective for me. It centres my breathing, helps me refocus and brings that head back in line with my body. I do Pilates at least twice a week, and it is by far the best thing that I do for my mind and body.

When Carol first arrived at The Pilates Centre, she wanted the answer to her chronic patterns immediately, so she could check it off her list. In time she realized that Pilates is a lifelong learning process with lifelong benefits, and students must approach – and practise – its method with that commitment in mind.

Through evaluation at The Pilates Centre, Carol learned that her forward head posture is the result of improper alignment of her feet and legs, the forward tilt of her pelvis, the consequent tightness of her hip flexors and lower back and the weakness of her abdominals. Using Pilates, she has straightened her leg and ankle alignment, elongated her hip flexors and lower back and strengthened her abdominal muscles. These changes have enabled her to lengthen and align her spine, ribcage and shoulder girdle, open her chest and settle her head in its proper uplifted position on top of her spine. Today, Carol has a sense of unlimited energy – she rides her bike, takes long walks and is considering early retirement so she can take advantage of her enthusiasm for life.

Pilates Works to Rehabilitate Shoulder Problems

Michael's case illustrates how lack of uniform development can cause problems stemming from one part of the body to be felt in another. Michael had a 'frozen' shoulder and lumbar instability. In evaluating his body mechanics, it became clear that his problems were actually caused by tight hamstrings.

How could tight hamstrings lead to a problem in the shoulder? When Michael flexed his spine, he couldn't access proper range of motion in his hip joints because of tight hamstrings. In time his lower back became overstretched, destabilizing his lumbar spine, for which he then compensated by protective 'tucking', which shortened his hamstrings even further. As a professional gardener, Michael performed this type of movement many times a day, bending over to pick things up, crouching to plant and adding an asymmetric load to his spine movements when shovelling earth.

The tight hamstrings and pelvic tuck threw Michael's spine out of proper alignment and disabled his Powerhouse. This in turn forced him to compensate by hypermobilizing his shoulder girdle to shovel soil and perform other activities. His shoulder joint became out of balance and stressed by the lack of stability in the shoulder girdle. The stress led to 'splinting' the joint, which eventually caused the capsule tissues to adhere to each other or become frozen.

Using the full range of Pilates equipment and exercises, The Pilates Centre worked with Michael towards the goal of uniform development. In his case, modified exercises focused on lengthening rather than shortening his hamstrings, correcting his specific pelvic and lumbar mechanics, strengthening his Powerhouse and teaching him to move his femur in his hip joint and his humerus in his shoulder joint. Pilates enabled him to flex his trunk correctly at the appropriate joints, alleviating the need to hypermobilize his shoulder girdle when reaching. His shoulder girdle developed stability and, consequently, his shoulder joint range of movement returned.

Pilates Is Movement Training, not Medicine

No matter how effective Pilates is when used in helping to heal injury and to bring the body back to health, it's essential to realize that Pilates is not a medical rehabilitation modality. The normal Pilates instructor certification process doesn't provide medical training, and your Pilates instructor isn't a doctor or a licensed physical therapist (although many licensed physical therapists have chosen to get their Pilates instructor certification). Pilates helps you achieve healing through movement and uses movement training to coordinate and uniformly develop your mind and body into a harmonious unity – one that's in sync with the waterfall of gravity.

> 'Self-confidence, poise [and] consciousness of possessing the power to accomplish our desires with renewed lively interest in life are the natural results of the practice of Contrology [Pilates].'
>
> Joseph Pilates, *Return to Life Through Contrology*

CHAPTER 21

Pursuing a Career in Pilates

I f you're reading this chapter, you have some interest in becoming a Pilates instructor. If you'd like to become a certified Pilates instructor in order to help people become and remain healthy, you're likely to find that it's one of the most rewarding, fulfilling careers anyone could hope for. Here you will learn more about the process and potential rewards of this exciting career.

Making the Decision to Pursue Pilates Certification

When you experience the profound benefits and amazing changes Pilates produces in your own body, you develop an abiding confidence in the Pilates methods. This is a strong foundation for a satisfying and meaningful professional life devoted to helping others achieve the same level of benefit you've enjoyed from doing Pilates. However, you need to approach the idea of certification soberly and seriously, to determine that it's the right choice – and the right time – for you.

Before you decide to embark on Pilates certification, consider your ability to deal with the inconveniences (and family-life disruption) of travel for training, the demands of study time, the impact of training on your income and the earnings potential for instructors in your chosen area. And don't underestimate the time it will take to become an accomplished student before you begin actual teacher training.

Preparation for Certification Takes Time

If you ask the Pilates 'elders ' – some of whom have been teaching Pilates for over 50 years – how long a person should study Pilates before becoming a teacher, all will recommend quite a few years' study. This lengthy learning curve may or may not be feasible for you, but the longer you remain a student of the method before entering a certification programme, the better prepared you'll be for becoming a good instructor.

Good instructors in any field need many years of experience in teaching their subject. Better instructors are those who have many years of practice before entering teaching, and draw upon those years in teaching their subject. And the best instructors are perpetual students: people who are in a continual process of learning, finding new ways to look at their subject, and developing their abilities. If you want to become one of the best Pilates instructors – the kind of teacher you would want to learn from – don't rush into teaching before you've studied a long time. True depth of knowledge comes only from experience and the willingness to remain a 'beginner'.

Pilates is an exact – and exacting – method. Pilates students need and deserve a well-seasoned instructor, someone who's been through the struggle, experienced the challenges and developed the rich understanding that accompanies the evolution of knowledge and skill. That evolution takes time. Studying Pilates involves learning the lessons your body has to teach – its habits, patterns, strengths and weaknesses – and those lessons unfold slowly.

Of course, years of experience bring many benefits to anyone who teaches Pilates. Here are just some of the bonuses of long-term training prior to entering a certification programme:

· You become an instructor with invaluable experience as a client. When you have firsthand knowledge of learning under good – and bad – instructors, you're better prepared to offer students effective, expert guidance.
· Extensive practice in the Pilates method gives you an opportunity to be sure you really love Pilates enough to commit to making it your career.
· The longer you study Pilates, the more uniformly fit you become, and you must be well on your way to uniform development to enter an instructor-training programme. During Pilates instructor training, you must perform every exercise at all levels of instruction (sometimes without a warm-up). If you aren't in top condition, you won't be able to accurately demonstrate the Pilates movements, and you might even injure yourself before your rigorous training is finished.

Would You Make a Good Instructor?

You have some years of experience practising the Pilates method, and you think you might like to become an instructor. But how do you know if you're a good candidate? Here are some questions that you should ask yourself:

- What skills, natural talents, background, education, experience and personality type do you already possess? Will any of them help you become a good teacher?
- Do you like to teach? Have you ever taught anything?
- Do you have any experience in other body-oriented techniques, such as dance, sports, yoga, martial arts, personal training or massage?
- Do you like to spend time with people, or are you an introvert?
- Are you patient when you explain processes and ideas, or do you want people to 'get it' quickly? Do the struggles of those trying to learn make you want to find new ways to help them, or do you just grow frustrated or bored with others' inability to learn?
- Do you feel comfortable working with people's bodies – putting your hands on them, lifting, pushing, watching them closely (see FIGURE 21-1)?

FIGURE 21-1

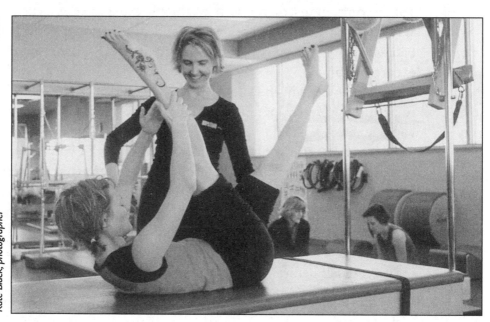

Kate Black, photographer

Teaching Pilates requires commitment, compassion, perseverance, energy, humour, kindness, focus, organization, discipline, physical and emotional endurance and an endless supply of patience. Learning to teach Pilates also requires a tremendous amount of time, energy and money, a high level of fitness, the humility necessary to be a beginner again and a willingness to take personal and professional risks.

Committing to Lifelong Learning

In particular, consider whether you possess the one quality that's essential to anyone choosing to become a Pilates instructor – your willingness to continue learning about Pilates every day of your life. Throughout this book, you've read that your body continues to evolve with each repetition, and that it won't be the same the next time you repeat any particular exercise. Those sentiments don't just apply to beginning-level students. Pilates is a process of lifetime evolution; your body's knowledge, awareness, experience and capabilities will continue to grow and change over a period of time.

Your teaching technique should evolve with each student and each lesson. The Pilates method of body conditioning is a continual process of growth, change, development and deepening understanding. If you are anxious to become an expert, someone who's achieved the peak Pilates learning experience and simply has nothing left to learn – no more questions to ask, no more advancements to achieve, no more mistakes to make – don't pursue a career in Pilates. A good Pilates instructor remains a student throughout his or her life.

Becoming a Pilates Instructor

There are several paths you can take to become an excellent Pilates instructor. Historically, Pilates teachers were apprenticed under the master or the master's protégés for many years. If you find a Pilates master willing to teach you, go for it; many of the best Pilates teachers working today learned this way.

However, most people don't have access to apprenticeship programmes with Pilates masters, and they need training programmes for their study. The good news is that a growing number of reputable certification programmes exist around the country and around the world.

The best way to become a truly effective Pilates teacher is to complete an extensive certification programme through a reputable, experienced, long-established school. A comprehensive certification programme will offer a systematic presentation of the Pilates method as a whole and, most importantly, a full and systematic presentation on how to teach Pilates to clients.

Acceptance into a reputable certification programme does *not* guarantee that you will receive Pilates certification. Reputable programmes have established, mandatory criteria for graduation with certification. You aren't looking for an attendance award; you want credible certification.

What to Look for in a Certification Programme

A reputable Pilates certification programme takes time, perhaps up to a year or more, and involves approximately 75 to 100 hours of lectures and 500 to 750 hours of practical work. Most reliable certification programmes also have established entrance requirements; entering students must pass a preliminary qualifications test or participate in a pre-certification programme to ensure that all candidates have achieved a certain level of Pilates fitness and a basic understanding of Pilates philosophy, methods and movement skills.

Here's a partial list of what a reputable certification programme might encompass:

· Training on all the Pilates equipment, to ensure that all certified instructors understand and appreciate the richness of the Pilates method – incorporating the equipment and mat work as interrelated parts of a comprehensive, integrated fitness system. Many Pilates instructors begin with mat-work certification before training using the full range of Pilates equipment.
· Training in the essential safety concerns surrounding the use of the equipment and the teaching of the exercises.
· Training in basic anatomy – to ensure that all certified instructors are able to identify major muscle groups, bones, organs and systems, and understand how they work.
· Techniques for appropriate modification of exercises for client-specific physical conditions, abilities and goals.

- Techniques for therapeutic applications of Pilates, used for physical rehabilitation of common complaints and injuries.
- Teaching and communications training, to ensure that certified instructors know the most effective ways to work with students of all body types, learning styles, ages, conditions and special needs.
- A required minimum number of hours in practical teaching training, so all graduates of the programme have a comprehensive understanding of (and plenty of time to practise) over 500 Pilates exercises and their modifications.
- A required minimum number of hours of instructor observation (see FIGURE 21-2), which allows future instructors to study the methods, teaching styles and techniques of experienced teachers at work in the studio, as they develop lesson structures, create good client relationships, adapt the method to individual needs and much more.
- A required minimum number of hours of personal lessons and workouts to continue to develop and maintain your Pilates fitness and skill level.

FIGURE 21-2:
Observing
Pilates
teachers
at work

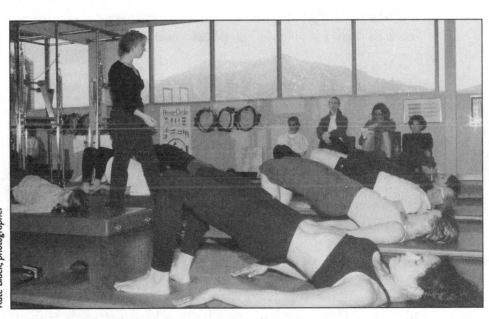

Kate Black, photographer

- Final written and practical examination covering the history, philosophy, pedagogy and technique of the Pilates method; case studies of possible client scenarios; anatomy; practical teaching technique; and an advanced level of personal proficiency in performing Pilates.

Choosing a Programme That's Right for You

Over the past ten years, certification programmes in the Pilates method have proliferated. One of your first considerations may be the lineage of the instructor or studio's Pilates training and its purity (how closely it adheres to the methods as taught by Joseph Pilates himself). Reread Chapter 2 for a deeper understanding of these distinctions. Some programmes adhere strictly to the classical lineage, others follow the personal developments of one particular elder, and some are hybrids of both approaches.

Pilates certification programmes come in all sizes. Like the differences between a small college and a large university, there can be pros and cons to each, and only you can decide which is best for you.

A number of programmes combine other movement theories and practices (such as Feldenkrais, Aston Patterning, yoga, Gyrotonics, physical therapy and so on) into an eclectic 'Pilates-based' blend. Just as with Pilates, each of these other practices requires a commitment to extensive study and exploration. Mixing them early in your training creates a lack of depth in the understanding of any one of them. It's best to fully immerse oneself in one discipline at a time to ensure a high level of understanding and eventual teaching ability.

Small Programmes

Programmes that accept fewer than a dozen trainees per year offer a number of advantages, including a low teacher-to-student ratio and an intimate environment in which all students begin and end their programme together as a homogeneous group. Small programmes can have drawbacks, too. Some might have only one teacher-trainer, whose personal ideas will influence the students' perspective on Pilates. Fewer trainers means fewer experienced teachers to observe, less flexibility in scheduling, a limited support structure, and fewer resources such as educational materials, advisors, financial aid, continuing education programmes and so on.

Large Programmes

Larger programmes generally offer more benefits, including larger studio space, more instructors, more equipment and more options for coursework, classes and personal workouts. You will probably have more opportunities for arranging observation sessions and apprenticeships, and a larger network of graduates to join and benefit from. Larger programmes also offer the variety of a large student body, with a variety of personalities, skills, ideas, goals and approaches. The larger organization can put more resources at your disposal, including support staff, advisors, educational materials, visiting instructors, special symposia, student discounts, financial aid and flexible payment schedules.

With all their advantages, large programmes can have their own set of drawbacks. You're likely to study in a classroom with a higher student-to-teacher ratio, with less personal attention. Being part of a larger student body, you may not experience the sense of togetherness present in a small group of trainees.

A Few Other Considerations

Here are a few other considerations in choosing a certification programme:

- Does the programme require teaching non-paying volunteer 'clients' on whom you can truly practise? Or does the programme encourage or even require you to teach paying clients before you have a comfortable amount of knowledge and experience under your belt? The longer you can be a student of teaching, the better.
- Does the school offer continuing education courses and require them for annual certification renewal?
- Does it offer travelling workshops that can come to you and your studio for continuing education or even part of your training?

· Does the programme offer job placement opportunities? Larger programmes often have a larger number of graduates with established studios or facilities that are looking to hire additional teachers.

Once you've graduated, you have several choices of venues in which to teach. For example, you can work for an established studio, health club or medical office, or open your own home studio or larger business. Each of these options has advantages and disadvantages, according to your own personal style and desires.

The Pilates Method Alliance

Your Pilates certification training and long years of practice will go far to make you a consummate Pilates professional. However, every Pilates student and instructor benefits from the ongoing guidance and knowledge of a professional organization. The Pilates Method Alliance (PMA), established in 2001, is a non-profit membership organization dedicated to raising the level of Pilates teaching worldwide, establishing an international board on testing standards and to creating 'an organization of qualified, dedicated professionals who share in Joseph H. Pilates's vision'. The PMA is a clearinghouse of information designed to provide facts for a better informed public.

The Pilates Method Alliance maintains a list of member studios and training programmes around the world, and is a good place to start in your exploration of the professional world of Pilates instruction. Visit their online site at www.pilatesmethodalliance.org. Anyone and everyone who is interested in the Pilates method, as a teacher, student or just plain enthusiast, will benefit by this organization.

'The mind, when housed within a healthful body, possesses a glorious sense of power.'

Joseph Pilates, letter to clients, 1939

Appendix A: Pilates Organizations

The following list is of Pilates organizations and training providers in the UK. In addition, contact any of them to find a local certified Pilates practitioner.

Polestar Pilates UK
98 Elmshurst Crescent
London N2 0LP
0870 246 0280
www.polestarpilates.co.uk

Pilates Umbrella
at Fitrooms
254–258 North End Road
London SW6 1NJ
0870 246 1800
www.pilatesumbrella.co.uk

Body Control
Body Control Pilates Studio
David Lloyd Club
Point West
118 Cromwell Road
London SW7
0207 244 8060
www.bodycontrol.co.uk

Alan Herdman Pilates
117 Homer Row
London W1H 4AP
0207 723 9953
www.alanherdmanpilates.co.uk

Stott Pilates
Quarry Court
Bell Lane
Cassington
Oxford OX9 4DS
0870 011 6530
www.stottpilates.com

Pilates Institute
Wimbourne House
151–155 New North Road
London N1 6TA
0207 253 3177
www.pilates-institute.com

PILATESfoundation UK Ltd
PO Box 36052
London SW16 1XQ
www.pilatesfoundation.com

Laban Pilates
Creekside
London SE8 3DZ
0208 691 8600
www.laban.org

Body Arts Sciences International
0207 228 1040
www.basipilates.com

Appendix B: Pilates Equipment

Books

Anatomy of Movement. By Blandine Calais-Germain. Eastland Press, Inc., 1993.

The Complete Writings of Joseph H. Pilates: Your Health and *Return to Life Through Contrology.* By Joseph H. Pilates. Compiled, edited, and revised by Sean P. Gallagher and Romana Kryzanowska. BainBridge Books, 2000.

The Pilates Body. By Brooke Siler. Broadway Books/Random House, Inc., 2000.

The Pilates Method of Body Conditioning: An Introduction to the Core Exercises. By Sean P. Gallagher and Romana Kryzanowska. BainBridge Books, 1999.

A Pilates Primer: The Millennium Edition, Return to Life Through Contrology and Your Health. By Joseph H. Pilates and William J. Miller. Presentation Dynamics, Inc., 2000.

Equipment

Balanced Body
Pilates equipment, accessories, videos, Gyrotonic
www.pilates.com

Pro Active
Complete online directory for UK fitness products
0870 848 4842
www.proactive-health.co.uk

Stott Pilates
Videos, equipment, accessories
0870 848 4843
www.stottpilates.com

Physical Company
Videos, accessories
01494 769222
www.physicalcompany.co.uk

Index